THE SEXUAL ~~REVOLUTION~~ HOLOCAUST

A Global Crisis

by Bridgette Heap
and Dr. John Sanford

DEDICATED TO
THE VICTIMS OF THE SEXUAL HOLOCAUST—
MAY THEIR COUNTLESS TEARS BE WASHED AWAY.

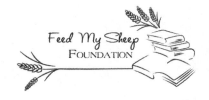

Feed My Sheep
FOUNDATION

The Sexual Holocaust: A Global Crisis.

ISBN# 978-0-9816316-6-0
Copyright © 2019

Published by FMS Publications, A Division of FMS Foundation, Inc., Canandaigua, NY USA.

Authors: Bridgette Heap and Dr. John Sanford
Technical Editor: Franzine Smith
Cover Design: Lorraine Larsen

CONTENTS

INTRODUCTION

W e are witnessing a profound change in the way
humans perceive and practice sexuality. Since
the beginning of written history, in most cultures,
sexual behaviors have been constrained, at some
level, by social norms. Such norms have typically fit
into the general parameters of family-based societies.
However, today much of the world is rejecting almost
all sexual constraints.

Most of the unrestrained sexual behaviors that are
becoming normalized today have been practiced in the
past—for example, in ancient Rome. Therefore, much
of the harm associated with unrestrained sexuality,
which we will describe, is not entirely new. However,
the harm associated with unrestrained sexuality has
never before been global, all-pervading, and widely
institutionalized. Many factors have contributed to the
globalization and normalization of these unrestrained
behaviors, including: (1) a wide-spread rejection
of faith-based morality; (2) the widespread use of
antibiotics; (3) the invention of effective contraceptives;
(4) the rise of the entertainment industry; and (5) the
feminist movement. These things contributed to *the
sexual revolution*. The sexual revolution has been
widely celebrated as a wonderful victory where *sexual
liberation* has triumphed over *sexual restraint*. Many
people now believe humanity is becoming freed from
all constraints, and this freedom is bringing joy and
personal fulfillment to billions of people.

Few people are aware of the profound *costs* of this "anything-goes" sexuality. It can be argued that the sexual revolution has caused more harmful consequences, more bondage, and more victims than any other human tragedy in history. Arguably, the sexual revolution has caused more human death and suffering than the Russian Revolution, the Chinese Cultural Revolution, World War I, World War II, or the Nazi Holocaust. All these tragedies were horrendous, but they were limited in space and time. However, the suffering associated with the sexual revolution is global in extent, continues to accelerate, and has no end in sight. It is in this light that we will refer to the sexual revolution and its diverse consequences as the *Sexual Holocaust*. **The Sexual Holocaust is a multi-dimensional global crisis stemming from unrestrained sexual behaviors that have resulted in profound harm to humanity.**

The term "holocaust" is most commonly used to describe the horror of the Nazi extermination of six million innocent Jewish people during World War II. The term "holocaust" is also used to describe *"destruction or slaughter on a mass scale, especially caused by fire or nuclear war."*[1] We do not wish to diminish the profound evil and suffering associated with the holocaust instituted by the Nazis; however, we wish to communicate the magnitude of the current crisis, as it is presently unfolding.

INTRODUCTION

During the Jewish Holocaust most of the world was silent. Some news spread of the horrors caused by the Nazis. However, people did not want to hear it. Neighboring nations did not want to get involved. America did not openly address the horror that was happening. People said the news leaking out was just hyperbole. The world closed their eyes and ears and let it happen. The same is happening today with unrestrained sexuality.

WHAT IS OUR GOAL?

This book is intended to be an overview. We have zoomed out to see the big picture. Our goal is not to judge or control, nor is it our goal to make judgements regarding sexual behaviors or to point blame. Instead, our goal is to *generate concern and empathy* for those being hurt by unrestrained sexual behaviors. We view human sexuality as a gift, but we will argue that unrestrained sexuality is extremely destructive. Our goal is to help people understand the magnitude of the Sexual Holocaust so that all caring and responsible people might work together to reduce the harm caused by unrestrained sexuality. The magnitude of the problem is such that we feel compelled to "sound the alarm." To do this, we will show how unrestrained sexuality negatively impacts all four dimensions of our humanity—the physical, the emotional, the social, and the spiritual. We will show that the four levels of harm are synergistic, with each amplifying the impact of the other. The result is escalating harm at every level.

We use numerous statistics in this overview, and we recognize that they will be obsolete in just a few years. Statistics always vary. However, this does not change the big picture. Because sexual issues are deeply private matters for most people, we are quite certain that most of the relevant statistics that are cited represent serious under-estimates. Our goal is not to write a technical report. Instead, our goal is to show the magnitude of the crisis.

We will begin at the simplest level by examining how unrestrained sexual behavior results in physical harm. We will then examine the other dimensions of the Sexual Holocaust, showing that at each additional level, there is increasing amplification of the problem.

CHAPTER 1

HARMFUL PHYSICAL CONSEQUENCES OF THE SEXUAL HOLOCAUST

The harmful physical consequences arising from the sexual revolution are the easiest harms to quantify and document. We can readily access a great deal of information based upon medical research and biomedical statistics. We wish to show how unrestrained sexual behaviors increase physical suffering on a global level. We will begin by looking at five specific examples of physical harm associated with the Sexual Holocaust: (1) Addiction, (2) Sexually-Transmitted Diseases, (3) Violence and Abuse, (4) Bondage and Slavery, and (5) Ubiquitous Abortion

ADDICTION

Pornography

A family physician,[2] whose name was kept confidential during an interview, confessed his addiction with pornography after being a user for over twenty years. He said it started innocently when he watched television in the fifties and sixties. Each week he experienced an "inexplicable thrill" when seeing scantily clad women on certain TV shows. When not watching, his imagination provided the same thrill away from the screen.

"My fantasy world grew. In it, I was either all-powerful or utterly powerless, usually bearing with stoic bravery some horrific injury, cared for by a legion of concerned females," he recalled. His fantasy world became a safe place for him to retreat to as he matured.

"I discovered masturbation at the same time I discovered soft-core pornography. It had an almost drug-like effect on me," he remembered. The physician recalled that at the age of 13 he discovered pornographic stores in the "big-city" that "displayed a cornucopia of sexual behavior." He compared the first time he read a sadomasochistic book to the first time a heroin user takes his first hit. He could not afford the books he wanted, so he began to steal them.

He recalled, "The pleasure I attained from reading these paperbacks and masturbating soon ruled my life. They created a safe place, a pleasurable place, one to which I could flee whenever I wanted." However, the more advanced stages of addiction were now in place. He believed that he was a bad person and that no one would love him if they knew his problem. To cope with these painful beliefs, he entered a helping profession and became a family physician.

Eventually, he met a woman who became his wife. He hid his addiction from her. With the invention of the Internet he was able to spend up to eight hours per day fueling his disturbing fantasies.

"The hours I wasted were taking their toll, and my life became increasingly unmanageable. I loathed the filth I created, promising each time it would be the last, and I lived in terror of being found out by my wife. I hated the lies that were necessary to cover up my detested secret life. I contemplated suicide, thinking that killing myself was preferable to living with the monster that was overpowering me."

Pornography is "printed or visual material containing the explicit description or display of sexual organs or activity, intended to stimulate erotic rather than aesthetic or emotional feelings."[3] Every imaginable type of pornography is now readily available. This includes: (1) sadism, which is "the tendency to derive pleasure, especially sexual gratification, from inflicting pain, suffering, or humiliation on others;" (2) masochism, which is "the tendency to derive pleasure, especially sexual gratification, from one's own pain or humiliation;" and (3) incestuous pornography, which displays sexual activity within families.

Pornography is everywhere we look. It is promoted, distributed, and normalized by respected main-stream corporate giants in the entertainment industry. It now accounts for a large part of all Internet traffic. It is even being promoted in university classrooms, such as at UCLA, UC Berkeley, and Bates College, to name a few.[4] So, how can such a pervasive, culturally accepted norm be causing so much harm? In this section, we will primarily look at the *physical* harms of pornography and the three types of victims associated with it.

The first group of victims are the users. Pornography physically harms the user's brain because of its addictive nature. Like all addictions, the brain is over-stimulated with endorphins. These endorphins can be easily triggered by viewing provocative visual images. Once the visual images have been seen, they can easily be recalled as mental images, once again over-stimulating the brain with endorphins. These endorphins are then powerfully amplified further by physical gratification. Like cocaine or other hard drugs, such endorphin-highs lose their potency over time—requiring higher doses (more and more extreme types of stimulation) to get the same high as before.

Pornography is being called "the new drug." A new non-religious, non-political organization is campaigning against pornography, and their slogan is "Fight the New Drug."[5] Pornography routinely results in hard-core addiction, and like all hard-core addictions, it changes how users think, how their brains work, and how they live. The need for higher doses takes users into increasingly dark and forbidden places—involving darker and darker fantasies such as sadomasochism, violence, and worse. Users who need unnatural or disturbing fantasies to get their endorphin-high will often eventually desire to act out those fantasies. Research shows that those who consume pornography are "more likely to support violence against women, to believe that women secretly enjoy being raped, and to actually be sexually aggressive in real life."[6]

The effects of pornography on the mind are similar to brain damage from illegal drugs. This is especially true for children. The effects of pornography on a developing child's brain is severe. According to the *Journal of the American Medical Association Psychiatry*, "pornography consumption is associated with decreased brain volume in the right striatum, decreased left striatum activation, and lower functional connectivity to the prefrontal cortex."[7]

Besides harming the brain through addiction, pornography also harms people's ability to cope in the real world. Pornography has increasingly become a coping or escaping mechanism. In one study, 73.8 percent of pornography consumers used pornography to alleviate stress, 70.8 percent used it to assuage boredom, and 53 percent used it to forget their daily problems.[8] Instead of finding healthy coping methods or long-term solutions to life's problems, individuals are seeking a quick fix through physical gratification associated with pornography. Pornography consumers find it increasingly difficult to cope with delayed gratification in every area of life because of pornography.[9]

The second group of victims are those in relationship with the user. Pornography not only harms the user, but it harms those who have a physical relationship with the user. Pornography decreases intimacy between partners and causes pornography consumers to need pornography in order to be aroused (instead of being aroused by their partners).[10] Many women find their partners impotent apart from pornography. An increasing number of therapists are counseling young healthy men suffering from impotency. The cause of their impotency is primarily pornography.[11] Users come to prefer a digital image over their actual partner or spouse. Kelly McDaniel, who is an author and licensed professional counselor in San Antonio, Texas, says that most pornography users she speaks with, "get to the point where they don't even like sex."[12] This can damage intimate physical relationships and be harmful to the one in the relationship with the user.

The third group of victims associated with pornography are specifically women and children. In 2010, a study, published in the journal *Violence Against Women*, looked at over 300 of the most popular pornographic scenes and found that 88.2% of those popular scenes included physical aggression and 48.7% included verbal aggression.[13] Of this aggression, 94.4% is directed towards women and girls.[14] As mentioned earlier, research shows that those who consume pornography are "more likely to support violence against women, to believe that women secretly enjoy being raped, and to actually be sexually aggressive in real life."[15] Soft-pornography (such as women's magazines and prime-time TV) is showing more and more explicit and violent images. Also, an *Esquire Magazine* headline read in February 2018 "Incest is the Fastest Growing Trend in Porn,"[16] making children vulnerable in what might seem to be stable households.

The use of pornography is ubiquitous and global. The percentage of men who regularly seek out pornography *several times a week* are: 63% of men ages 18-30, 38% of men ages 31-49, and 25% of men ages 50-68.[17] Many more seek it out less frequently. "Only 10 percent of men 25+ say they never seek out porn."[18] If these numbers reflect a broader reality, then the large majority of all males alive today may be presently using pornography, and up to 32% of all males could be addicted. Many men do not even know they are addicted because they have been bound to it since childhood and consider it a natural part of their life. They have never tried to be free of it. It is difficult to know the extent of addiction because people who have not tried to quit cannot know if they are addicted. If these numbers are correct, over 1 billion men may presently be addicted to pornography, with women quickly catching up.

For women, the percent that regularly seek out pornography is: 21% of women ages 18-30, 5% of women ages 31-49, and 0% of women ages 50-68.[19] Though fewer women seek pornography than men, 17% of women describe themselves as addicted to pornography.[20] We suspect these numbers are understated due to the reluctance of most people to fully admit the extent of their viewing and the extent of their addiction.

Pornography is affecting both religious and secular populations alike. For example, studies show that "60% of Christian men, and 40% of Christian women struggle with porn."[21] There are many factors that contribute to the frequency of pornography use, including age, gender, and faith commitments. A survey from the Barna group shows how these factors influence the frequency of pornography use in the United States (see Appendix 1, Figure 1).[22] According to the survey, women consume pornography less than men. Older generations consume pornography less than younger generations. Finally, practicing Christians consume pornography less than non-practicing Christians.

Surprisingly, adult males are not the leading consumers of pornography. "The largest consumer of internet pornography is 12 to 17-year-olds."[23] Studies also show that "64% of young people, ages 13-24, actively seek out pornography weekly or more often."[24] Even pre-teen children are actively consuming pornography. *"Internal intelligence from Bitdefender's parental control feature revealed that the under-10 age group is now accounting for one in 10 of the visitors to porn video sites* (emphasis added)."[25] According to the *British Journal of School Nursing*, "children under 10 now account for 22% of online porn consumption under 18."[26] The average age of first viewing is 11 years old and is still dropping.[27] This means roughly 50% of first-time-viewers are children under 11 years old. Studies show that "almost 90 percent of college age young men and 30 percent of the young women view pornography."[28]

It is no mystery why pornography consumption is so prevalent. Pornography is easily accessible. More than 4.6 billion hours of pornography were consumed on one leading pornography website alone in the year 2016.[29] In an article about how big pornography sites really are, Sebastian Anthony explains that they make up 30% of the Internet traffic. Such sites are bigger than regular movie sites, such as Hulu.[30] Seventy percent of "porn viewing occurs during normal business hours"[31] and, more surprisingly, is often viewed in public. In a study done with 15,000 global respondents, one in six admitted to watching pornography on a public network or other public server.[32] In 2017, Norton by Symantec conducted a global survey, which likewise showed that one in six people admit to watching pornography publicly in places like hotels and Airbnb's, cafes and restaurants, airports, at work, on the street, in train and bus stations, and in public restrooms.[33] Almost three-quarters of young adults, about 71%, and half of teens "come across what they consider to be porn at least once a month, whether they are seeking it or not."[34]

The harmful consequences of pornography continue to increase because individuals are not warning each other about the effects of pornography. Studies show that 87 percent of individuals say "that no one in their lives is helping them avoid pornography."[35] Fifty-four percent of those could not "even think of anyone who could help them."[36] Sadly, "the United States is a top consumer of both illegal child pornography and obscene pornography,"[37] and the mentality today is that not recycling is more immoral than viewing pornography.[38]

Our discussion begins with pornography because it is the primary force driving all types of unrestrained sexual behavior. However, pornography is not the only addiction related to unrestrained sexual behaviors. Sexual behaviors are closely linked with drug and alcohol use. Most drug addicts use more than one harmful substance, and logically, this applies to "the new drug" (pornography). Pornography addicts seek other drugs to enhance their experience. Addictions are complex and overlapping.

Drugs and Alcohol

Drug and alcohol addictions are directly related to prostitution and porn-acting. Sometimes drug and alcohol use may just be part of the lifestyle of a prostitute or a porn-star. However, drugs are often used to ease the emotional pain associated with these unrestrained sexual lifestyles, which will often lead to complex addictions involving both drugs and sex. People with such lifestyles then need to maintain their sexual lifestyle to help fund their other addictions, creating a vicious cycle.

Sex-trafficking is also often associated with drugs. Pimps initiate and feed drug addictions to ensure their trafficked victims remain dependent on them.[39] Drug addiction causes serious physical issues, but it also creates the emotional connection between the pimps and their victims. Victims want and need the drugs because it helps reduce the physical and emotional pain of being sexually exploited. The pimps provide the drugs for the purpose of control.

Several studies have shown that 61-64% of sexual "hookups" followed alcohol consumption and more than half of those sexual encounters occurred directly because of alcohol use.[40] Alcohol consumption has been linked to a variety of types of sexual hookups, showing that those who have consumed greater amounts of alcohol did more sexually extreme acts, while those who consumed less, did less. In her book, *American Hookup*, Dr. Lisa Wade, Associate Professor of Sociology, explains that drinking is a vital part of hooking-up. In fact, it is part of the "pregame." Hooking-up begins with drinking *before* going out for the evening to meet someone. Arriving at parties already in a state of intoxication is part of the culture.[41]

The *American Psychological Association* commented in a report on the hookup culture that "alcohol may also serve as an excuse, purposely consumed as a strategy to protect the self from having to justify hookup behavior later."[42] Testimonies shared with Dr. Wade by sorority students confirms the association of drinking with sexual activities. Sorority members, who were asked to remain sober during parties to help facilitate the party, were disgusted by what they saw. However, they admitted that when intoxicated, all these behaviors no longer seemed disgusting.[43]

In summary, unrestrained sexual behavior can lead to addiction. Pornography of every imaginable type is now readily available to almost any adult or child on the planet. As a consequence, our world is now hyper-sexualized to an extent that exceeds ancient Rome. A large fraction of humanity is now addicted to pornography and supplemental drugs—creating unspeakable physical harm. There is a leading movement in western culture today to normalize pornography use and to reduce feelings of guilt associated with its use. Naomi Wolff, a leading feminist and progressivist author asks "But does all this sexual imagery in the air mean that sex has been liberated?" She continues,

"—or is it the case that the relationship between the multi-billion-dollar porn industry, compulsiveness, and sexual appetite has become like the relationship between agribusiness, processed foods, supersize portions, and obesity? If your appetite is stimulated and fed by poor-quality material, it takes more junk to fill you up. People are not closer because of porn but further apart; people are not more turned on in their daily lives but less so."[44]

Responsible individuals need to become aware of the incredible cost of unrestrained sexual behaviors and the need to promote sexual responsibility. Pornography does not satisfy sexual desires, instead it creates unnatural, dehumanizing, and unquenchable lusts. We will further discuss pornography in the "Emotional Harms" section.

SEXUALLY-TRANSMITTED DISEASE (STD)

AIDS

When Teddy was eleven, her mother lay on a bed, unable to attend to the children, work, or even care for herself. Teddy cooked the food, washed the clothes, and boiled herbs to soothe her mother's aches. It would not be long before her mother would be dead, along with her father.

"I am suffering from AIDS, Teddy," her mother would say. Teddy wished her mother would explain how she contracted the disease and how Teddy and the other children could stay safe, but her mother never did. When she died, the children began to go hungry.

Family members and neighbors stole from them and ridiculed them "They are probably infected too!"[45]

AIDS, which stands for *acquired immunodeficiency syndrome*, is the advanced phase of infection by the virus called HIV. HIV stands for *human immunodeficiency virus* and is a virus that attacks the immune system. Once the immune system is weakened, individuals also become more susceptible to other diseases. Antiretroviral treatment/therapy (ART) can prolong life, slow symptoms, and reduce transmission to others. However, there is still no widely available cure for HIV. With ART treatment, HIV infected individuals are living longer. However, without treatment, the disease still consistently progresses to its final stage, AIDS. When this happens, victims become increasingly disabled and die.[46] Even with treatment, it is not clear that the progression of the disease will be fully halted.

There are more than 40 antiviral drugs that have been approved to help treat HIV. Those who have been infected will have to take two or more of these drugs every day for the rest of their lives to slow the progression of the disease.[47] The side effects of these drugs can be severe[48] and make ART a difficult treatment to live with. However, strict adherence to daily dosages are required, otherwise the HIV virus may become resistant to the drugs and can once again be transmitted. Widespread resistance of HIV to these drugs could be catastrophic.

Over twenty-five million people living in Africa are infected with HIV.[49] In many African countries, 10-20% of the people are infected with HIV. However, HIV is not just devastating Africa, but is a global crisis. In 2018, 37.9 million people were infected with AIDS worldwide.[50] As of 2017, 25% of those infected were not even aware they were infected.[51] It is estimated that there are 5,000 global, new infections that occurred *daily*.[52] In 2018, there were 770,000 AIDS-related deaths worldwide.

Sexually-Transmitted Diseases in General

HIV is not the only incurable sexually-transmitted disease (STD). Of the eight most prevalent sexually-transmitted diseases, only half are curable. Chlamydia, gonorrhea and syphilis are bacteria-based infections and can be cured with antibiotics. Antibiotics can also be used to cure trichomoniasis, a parasite-based infection. However, hepatitis B, herpes simplex virus (HSV-2), and human papillomavirus (HPV) are STDs that are non-curable viruses, similar to HIV.[53] This means that those who are infected with these diseases will live with them for the rest of their lives. The symptoms these individuals will suffer include: pelvic inflammatory disease, infertility, tubal or ectopic pregnancy, cervical cancer, warts, and infections in mucous membranes throughout the body.[54]

Individuals may have a sexually transmitted infection (STI), which means they are infected with a virus, but may not yet show symptoms. Only after the symptoms appear, can they be diagnosed with an STD.[55] The Center for Disease Control and Prevention (CDC) estimates that in the United States 51% of those infected with HIV between the ages 13-24 do not know they are infected.[56] Individuals may be infected but may not know they are, because not everyone gets tested for infection and because symptoms may not appear for many years. Many infected women do not show symptoms but may have serious physical complications that are attributed to other health issues.[57] STDs can also be passed down to the next generation. Children born to STD-infected mothers can inherit the same disease with all its harmful effects. Equally disturbing is that babies born to mothers with an STD may be born with perinatal and congenital complications.[58]

The 2019 report from the World Health Organization, indicates that in the previous year over a billion people had one or more STDs.[59] The report says that "more than 1 million sexually transmitted infections (STIs) are acquired every day worldwide."[60] It also reports that "there were an estimated 376 million new infections with 1 of 4 STIs: chlamydia, gonorrhea, syphilis and trichomoniasis."[61] WHO estimates that over 500 million people worldwide have HSV-2 (genital herpes).[62] "More than 290 million women have a human papillomavirus (HPV) infection."[63]All this adds up to more than 1 billion infections in a single year.

The CDC estimates "that undiagnosed STIs cause 24,000 women to become infertile each year."[64] In 2016, over 988,000 pregnant women were infected with syphilis. This resulted in approximately 350,000 adverse birth outcomes, including stillbirths.[65] STDs are also creating a large number of orphans who need to be cared for. Teddy (see above) is just one of the 16.6 million orphans alive today who have lost their parents to an STD.[66]

Some might think that money and education will reverse this enormous STD problem. However, these diseases are primarily spreading because sexual behaviors are not being restrained. Many people are exposed to STDs because they are addicted, coerced, seduced, act compulsively, or are simply irresponsible. These types of behaviors do not go away simply through better education. The 2019 report from UNAIDS said that "in 2018, more than half of all new HIV infections were among key populations," such as sex workers, people who use drugs, men who have sex with men, transgender people, prisoners, and the partners of these people.[67] Clearly, key populations have a high-risk of exposure to STDs. Furthermore, many young adults across the globe are also at great risk because of the promiscuous hookup culture. Between 60 and 80% of western college students participate in the hookup culture.[68] "It is estimated that one in four college students will contract an STD during their time at school. In the larger population, this works out to 50% of people get an STD at some time in their life."[69] Because few realize the extent of the problem, the majority of students do not even ask if their partner is infected, and often do not bother to have protected sex. Though ART drugs and antibiotics are helping to decrease STD symptoms, diseases continue to spread.

Many people are trusting that antibiotics and antiviral drugs can be their "plan B." They do not understand that many STDs are simply not curable. STDs that are presently curable may soon become incurable, due to drug-resistant STDs arising from reckless, illegal, and prophylactic use of antibiotics. The 2019 WHO report indicated grave concern due to "...high rates of quinolone resistance, increasing azithromycin resistance and emerging resistance to extended-spectrum cephalosporins. Drug resistance, especially for gonorrhea, is a major threat..."[70] If widespread antibiotic resistance develops, the STDs that we can now readily control with antibiotics (gonorrhea and syphilis) may once again become deadly.

People are devastated when they are diagnosed with an incurable STD and realize they will have it the rest of their life. Even more tragic is the harm caused by unrestrained sexual behaviors that cause STDs to be passed on to either children or other loved ones. Such profound suffering is the consequence of "anything-goes" sexuality. Responsible individuals are starting to see that the price of this type of liberated sexuality is simply too high.

Violence and Abuse

"Her name was Jyoti Singh," a mother said to an emotionally charged crowd in India.[71] Jyoti was 23 and studying physiotherapy. On December 16, 2012 she was brutally gang-raped by six men on a moving bus in New Delhi.[72] She had been stabbed with a metal rod that punctured her colon and had been dumped on the street naked and bleeding. After two hours she was found by the police. Her attackers were identified in part by the bite marks they left on her body. Two weeks later, she died in the hospital from her wounds.[73]

Jyoti Singh was the victim of a gang rape. Other forms of rape include acquaintance rape, statutory rape, partner rape, and incest.[74] Victims who are raped often suffer horrible physical harm. Their bodies and their reproductive organs can be severely damaged during rape. As mentioned earlier, rape or abuse victims are also at risk of being infected by sexually-transmitted diseases (STDs). STDs can produce serious long-term physical pain for victims. Female rape victims also often have unwanted pregnancies and, therefore, suffer through the pain of either an abortion or the pain of childbirth. A study conducted in 1993 showed that for women who were of reproductive age, one of the effects of rape and domestic violence was a reduced life span of one to five years.[75]

It is not just an unfortunate few that suffer from sexual violence and abuse. This is a global concern. Nearly one in five women and one in thirty-eight men in the United States have reported experiencing rape or attempted rape at some time in their lives.[76] However, South Africa has the highest recorded account of rape of any country. The number of reported accounts of rape increased from 2017 to 2018 with an average of 114 rapes recorded by the police each day.[77] It is estimated that "35% of women globally have experienced physical or sexual violence."[78] This is over a billion women. A 2006 study says that in Canada, every minute one woman is sexually assaulted.[79] The World Health Organization (WHO) estimates that "1 in 3 (35%) women worldwide have experienced either physical and/or sexual intimate partner violence or non-partner sexual violence in their lifetime."[80] Also according to the WHO, as many as 38% of all global murders of women are committed by intimate partners.[81]

Children are also suffering sexual violence and abuse. According to the organization *Invisible Children*, "1 in 4 girls and 1 in 6 boys will be sexually abused before they turn 18 years old." This means, on average, about 20% of all children are being abused. This means that over time the number of abused children greatly exceeds 1 billion.

Children who are being sexually abused may exhibit many symptoms. These include depression and/or withdrawal from others, anxiety, nervousness (especially about being alone), fear of people who remind them of their abuser, hyper-vigilance, anger, change in appetite and/or eating disorders, suicidal and/ or other self-harming behaviors, low self-esteem and feelings of worthlessness, sleep problems including nightmares, trouble concentrating, confusion, unusual aggressiveness, lack of trust, secretiveness, excessive compliance, refusal to go to school, abnormal interest in anything of a sexual nature, complaints of something wrong in the genital area, or seductive behaviors.[82] The trauma of sexual abuse can last into adulthood. Many adults who were victims as children try to compensate for their abuse by aspiring to gain successful careers in order to find self-worth. Addiction to drugs, alcohol, pornography or other escapes become prominent coping mechanisms. Statistics show that victims of sexual assault and rape are likely to become rapists and assaulters themselves. They abuse or manipulate people in order to stay in control. As mentioned earlier, this is an example of the amplifying affect, which multiplies the physical harm caused by unrestrained sexual behaviors. The next generation will witness an unprecedented number of people suffering from sexual violence and abuse. This will include more than a billion women and a billion children.

Although sexual violence is not new, it is significantly amplified by pornography and the entertainment industry, and is, therefore, now being normalized globally. These media platforms are putting women and children at increased risk of violence and abuse.

The Sexual Holocaust

It is clear that the emerging "anything-goes" sexuality is not liberating women. In fact, it seems to be doing the opposite. The Sexual Holocaust has fundamentally dehumanized people—especially women and children—by making them objects of entertainment and pleasure. All responsible people across the world need to become aware of the incredible cost of unrestrained sexuality and the need to promote sexual responsibility.

Slavery and Bondage

Tonya[83] (pseudonym) knew Eddie (pseudonym) for a few years on and off. She had been friends with his step-daughter when she was 13. They had flirted with each other from time to time, but nothing happened until they reconnected in a bar when Tonya was 15. Tonya had become a runaway within those years and Eddie was no longer married. Tonya began to stay with Eddie, taking care of his children, cleaning, and cooking. They had a physical relationship with each other.

One night, when they went to a party with drugs and alcohol, Eddie asked Tonya to sleep with a man for money. At first she refused, but after half an hour of pressure and coaxing, Eddie convinced Tonya to just try it this once. This one-time affair became a regular routine. Eddie found "suitors" for Tonya, and Tonya agreed because she believed she loved Eddie.

In an interview Tonya recalls, "Being able to sleep with that many people and live with myself and get up every day and keep doing it and just lying there being helpless was so hard." Eventually, the Grand Prairie, Texas police department received a tip about Eddie's crimes, and he was arrested.

There are two major forms of human trafficking: labor trafficking and sex trafficking.[84] In this overview, we will discuss sex trafficking. "Sex trafficking is the crime of using force, fraud or coercion to induce another individual to perform commercial sex. Common types include escort services, pornography, illicit massage businesses, brothels, and outdoor solicitation."[85]

Individuals can become enslaved in various ways. Sometimes individuals are physically captured, bonded, and forced to perform sexual acts. Sometimes, they are tricked by a person offering to help them financially. They may be told they are getting a decent job, only to learn they have been deceived and are expected to work as a prostitute or sex-slave, often with no pay. Others, like Tonya, are persuaded or threatened by family members or those they love to subject themselves to sexual acts. Children may even be willingly handed over to traffickers by parents who cannot afford to keep them.[86]

Whatever the reasons may be for how individuals end up in slavery, the result is horrifying. Like rape victims, individuals in sexual bondage experience similar consequences, including: physical pain, damage to their body, exposure to STDs, and potential unwanted pregnancies. Prostitutes, though not always forced to have sexual intercourse, are asked to perform sexual acts that can be painful and degrading. Prostitutes and trafficked sex-workers are often physically abused.

It is important to note that trafficked victims often become enslaved to their work for numerous reasons. Some find it necessary to work more in order to make ends meet or to pay a debt. Some believe they cannot escape because they would not be able to find another form of employment if they left. Some individuals are given drugs to create a physical addiction, as mentioned in the "Addiction" section above.

There are 24.9 million people trafficked worldwide and more than half of these people are sexually exploited.[87] Sex trafficking does not just happen in third world countries where "mail-order brides" are common and girls as young as 13 are given in "marriage." Sex-trafficking is plaguing prosperous nations as well. In 2015, the Department of Homeland Security in the United States arrested more than 1,400 criminals on human trafficking offenses.[88] At least one in five men in America have solicited a prostitute. This is an example of the amplifying effect mentioned earlier. Men who solicit prostitutes are more likely to have been molested as children than those who do not solicit prostitutes. We see the unrestrained sexual behavior of molestation causing harmful consequences in these men's lives. In return, these men are more likely to have unrestrained sexual behaviors, like hiring a prostitute, which in turn, perpetuates the consequence of bondage in someone else's life. These men often force women into sexual acts.[89]

It is estimated that there are forty to forty-two million prostitutes worldwide.[90] "The average age at which girls first become victims of prostitution is 12 to 14 years old, and the average age for boys is 11 to 13 years old."[91] The majority of prostitutes become involved in sex-trade because they either ran away from parents when teenagers and needed a job, or they were sexually exploited as children. This is another example of the amplifying effect. The physical suffering in a child's life, caused by someone's unrestrained sexual behavior, has caused many of them to engage in further unrestrained sexual behaviors, such as prostitution. Every year, "traffickers exploit one million children in the commercial sex trade."[92]

Supporters of the sexual revolution think that the result is the advancement of *free love*; however, the millions of people in bondage would not call this *free*. They are paying the price for unrestrained sexuality—and the price is too high. Responsible people need to help sound the alarm about the Sexual Holocaust.

UBIQUITOUS ABORTION

In South Korea, a young woman decided to get an abortion at two months along. Her procedure was a curettage abortion, which detaches the fetus from the walls of the uterus, typically through suction or loop shaped tools which scrape the uterus lining. A few months later, this woman realized she was still pregnant. The abortion had failed. She decided to give birth to the baby and give it up for adoption. A family in the United States adopted the baby and named him Josiah Presley.

Today, Josiah speaks about induced abortion and the harms it causes. An induced abortion is "an abortion that is brought about intentionally," not spontaneously, such as a miscarriage.[93] Josiah describes one type of induced abortion procedure. "A curettage abortion is a type of abortion where the doctor goes into the mother's womb and basically rips the baby apart and brings them out in pieces, and that's actually why we think that I'm probably missing an arm today." Josiah was otherwise a completely healthy baby, but stands as a testament to the physical harm caused by abortion.[94]

The ongoing debate of when a human fetus becomes human, has human value, or has human rights will not be resolved in the near future. Regardless of exactly when an embryo becomes human, there is medical research that shows that induced abortions cause more physical harm than any other topic we have discussed so far.

In this section, we will describe three types of induced abortion and the physical harms they can cause the mother and/or the fetus. Next, we will describe some misconceptions of induced abortion. Finally, we will explain why induced abortions are a global concern and why they are causing more physical harm than any other topic we have discussed so far. From this point forward, we will simply refer to induced abortions as abortions. We will not be discussing miscarriages or stillbirths, which arise apart from human will.

There are several types of abortions: aspiration abortion (given within the first trimester), dilation and evacuation (given during the second trimester), and induction abortion (given during the third trimester).[95] Scientists and doctors in the fields have shown that through these various types of abortions, both the mothers and fetuses feel pain. Aspiration abortions forcibly suck the fetus out of the uterus. This can cause women extreme pain, nausea, excessive bleeding, and may lead to further complications with future pregnancies.[96] According to scientific research, a fetus's nervous system is formed by four weeks.[97] By 8 weeks, neural pathways in the fetus's brain are forming. At this point, a woman cannot feel the fetus, and may have just discovered the pregnancy. A fetus's reflexes have already developed at this stage as well. By 10 weeks, scientists say it is possible for a fetus to feel pain in the womb. It is at this point that an aspiration abortion would be performed.

Dilation and Evacuation abortions, done during the second trimester, are increasingly risky for the mother. The fetus, which can feel pain throughout its body at this point and can survive outside the mother's womb if given support, is torn apart by the physician and removed piece by piece. It is then reassembled to make sure all pieces of the fetus were extracted. Broken bones from the fetus are a serious risk to the mother because they can puncture her uterus and damage her reproductive organs. This risk also applies to her bowels, bladder, and rectum. At this stage, the placenta is tightly adhered to the uterus wall and considerable scraping is necessary to detach it from the mother.[98]

Induction abortion, performed during the third trimester, has the greatest risks for the mother and fetus. A long needle full of a lethal chemical is injected into the fetus through the mother's abdomen or vagina. Laminaria sticks are inserted into the mother to begin dilating the cervix. The mother leaves the clinic and typically waits 2-3 days until she is dilated. Upon returning to the clinic, an ultrasound test is given to see if the fetus is still alive. If so, it is given another dose of the lethal chemical. The mother tries to make it to the clinic upon having contractions, but if not, she delivers at home, typically over a toilet. If the fetus does not come out whole, it becomes a dilation and evacuation procedure and is removed piece by piece. These late-term abortions cause the most pain and risks for the mothers and the fetuses. The mothers will experience forced contractions and labor, which may last days. Complications increase with second pregnancies because of this procedure. These procedures also cause the most pain for the fetus. At this stage in development, the baby can fully survive outside the womb. Medical researchers have shown that fetuses may even experience more pain within the womb than after birth. Because the lethal doses of chemicals meant to kill the baby do not always work immediately, a fetus can suffer over several days, dying slowly.[99]

Even women who have undergone a clinically safe abortion can still suffer serious side-effects. After an abortion, women can suffer from any number of physical complications, including "hemorrhage requiring transfusion, perforation of the uterus, cardiac arrest, endotoxic shock, major unintended surgery, infection resulting in hospitalization, convulsions, undiagnosed ectopic (tubal) pregnancy, cervical laceration, and uterine rupture."[100] However, unsafe abortions are common. Nearly half of all abortions are performed without a trained medical technician and in an unsafe medical environment. This practice is one of the leading causes of life-long medical complications in women and maternal mortalities, claiming nearly 70,000 women a year.[101]

There are misconceptions surrounding abortion. Many argue that abortions are (1) safe, (2) the mother's choice, (3) a resource for rape victims who suffer from unwanted pregnancies, (4) sometimes required for the mother's health, and (5) sometimes required because the fetus is inviable. We have already discussed how abortions are not necessarily safe for either the mother or the fetus, even in a safe, sterile medical environment with trained professions. Now, we will look at the other misconceptions surrounding abortion.

Abortion is often not the mother's choice. Most women admit that they did not want to abort their babies. They had an abortion simply because they felt pressured to have one. They give the following reasons for their abortions: (1) their family won't support them; (2) their boyfriends won't stay with them; (3) they are told they are not ready to raise a child; or (4) they are told they will not enjoy life struggling to raise a child. Many women are pressured or coerced into having an abortion and are reassured that the procedure is safe. If such women felt free to choose, and they knew they would be supported with resources that empower them, then many more might make decisions that do not risk harm to their bodies and to the bodies of their babies.

Many people support abortions in sympathy for women who had unintended pregnancies by rape. However, abortions due to rape represent special cases, which are rare. Abortions due to rape and incest combined only account for 1.5% of abortions being performed globally today.[102] Medically speaking, women who are pregnant due to rape are more vulnerable to possible negative abortion outcomes. The damage already done to their body by rape can put them at greater physical risk during an abortion, and they are at a higher emotional risk. A study conducted showed that those who had "pre-existing experience of trauma" or "past or present sexual, physical, or emotional abuse" were at a higher risk for "negative post-abortion psychological adjustment."[103] Abortions are, therefore, not the safest choice for rape victims.

Many people support abortions out of concern for the mother's health. As in the case with rape, these instances are special cases, which are rare. Similarly, people support abortion out of concern for fetal health issues. Again, these are special cases that are rare. In 2004, the Guttmacher Institute surveyed women in the United States who had had an abortion. Less than 0.5% said they had an abortion because of rape. About 3% said they had an abortion because of fetal health issues. About 4% said they had an abortion because of their own personal health issues.[104] According to the WHO, health professionals today say that most of the complications due to pregnancy that lead to maternal mortality "are preventable or treatable."[105]

The survey from Guttmacher Institute showed that 92% of participants gave the following reasons for having an abortion: would interfere with education or career, not mature enough to raise a child, didn't want to be a single mother, done having children, can't afford a baby, or not ready for a child.[106]

We chose to discuss abortion last because global abortion rates eclipse all other types of death associated with lack of sexual restraint. In fact, *global abortion rates eclipse all other causes of death* (see Appendix 1, Figure 2). Every year there are roughly 50 million abortions globally. Abortions claim more lives every year than the top ten leading causes of death *combined*. While there are about 50 million abortions globally per year, there are "only" 34 million deaths globally due to heart disease, stroke, respiratory infections, COPD, lung cancer, diabetes, Alzheimer's/dementia, diarrheal disease, tuberculosis, and road accidents *combined*.[107] In the United States, the CDC reported that for every 1,000 live births, there were 188 abortions. This means Americans killed more than 18% of those who would have been born in the year 2015. In some parts of the world, the rate is much higher. Since 1980, at least one and a half billion developing humans have been intentionally killed worldwide.[108] In addition to these 1.5 billion aborted babies, there have been countless women negatively impacted by abortions. Regardless of one's perspective on the humanity of the developing new life, it is clear that abortions are impacting the world to a far greater extent than anything else that we will address.

The vast majority of abortions are the result of unrestrained sexual behaviors. The physical cost of abortion is the obvious physical harm to countless unborn babies and countless mothers.

PHYSICAL CONSEQUENCES

PHYSICAL HARM SUMMARY

The Sexual Holocaust is globally creating immeasurable physical harm to countless people, year in and year out. This is impacting most families and a large part of the human race. This tragic problem continues to get worse. However, these physical harms are eclipsed by the other types of harm that are arising due to the Sexual Holocaust. In the following sections, we will look at the emotional, social, and spiritual harms of the Sexual Holocaust.

CHAPTER 2

HARMFUL EMOTIONAL CONSEQUENCES OF THE SEXUAL HOLOCAUST

We all experience emotional pain—it is part of life. However, the emotional pain associated with the Sexual Holocaust is long-lasting, life-shattering, and can be life-threatening. It should be obvious that the physical harms that arise from unrestrained sexual behaviors will almost always bring with them serious emotional harms. What may not be so obvious is that the emotional harm caused by unrestrained sexual behaviors can far exceed the physical harm, both in severity and in duration.

In this chapter, we will first take a look at the relationship between the physical harms of the previous chapter and emotional harms caused by unrestrained sexual behaviors. Then, we will examine four specific examples of emotional harm caused by the Sexual Holocaust, which are deeper and longer lasting than the physical harm seen in the previous section: (1) Loneliness, (2) Rejection, (3) Depression, and (4) Suicide.

THE RELATIONSHIP BETWEEN
PHYSICAL AND EMOTIONAL HARMS

The Emotional Cost of Addiction

Just as we started with pornography in the previous section, we will start with it again. Pornography use leads to guilt, shame, and loneliness. However, there is a leading movement in western culture today to normalize pornography use and to reduce the feeling of guilt associated with its use. There are many websites devoted to helping pornography addicts feel better about using pornography. These websites try to justify pornography while trying to ease people's conscience. They refuse to address the real issue—unrestrained sexuality. Over time, many users may lose the negative emotional feelings they once had when consuming pornography. This is dangerous because it teaches individuals to simply set aside their consciences for temporary pleasure. Suppressing the negative emotions and the appropriate sense of guilt associated with pornography use contributes to addiction, disease, violence, bondage, and death.

Pornography has a deep emotional effect on men and women. It effects their identity and their sense of self-worth. Seeking ways to enhance one's sex-appeal becomes an unhealthy compulsion for many, perhaps most, pornography viewers. As people view pornography, they learn to compare their bodies to those they see on the screen.

An esthetician, specializing in hair removal, admitted that she was disturbed that the most common question she received from her female clients when performing bikini/Brazilian services was "Does it look normal down there? Am I normal?" She was concerned, first, that most women of all ages did not know what normal female genitalia should look like, and second, that they were not asking their medical doctors for advice in this area.[109] It is not surprising to see why women are uncomfortable with their own bodies.

When women see surgically enhanced women in pornographic films, they question what is "normal" and even what is beautiful and appealing. Labiaplasty is an elective, cosmetic surgery done by women to change the size or shape of their labia minora by trimming. "Taken a step further, a procedure called 'The Barbie' amputates the entire labia minora, in order to make a woman's labia look smooth like a plastic doll."[110] Today, the leading cosmetic trend among women and girls is elective genital reconstruction surgery.[111] These surgeries, however, are not correcting unhealthy bodies. Instead, these surgeries are damaging healthy bodies just to produce a certain sex appeal. Because of porn stars, normal, healthy women are insecure with their own anatomy.

Pornography makes women feel inadequate and worthless. Naomi Wolf writes on the topic:

> "The young women who talk to me on campuses about the effect of pornography on their intimate lives speak of feeling that they can never measure up, that they can never ask for what they want; and that if they do not offer what porn offers, they cannot expect to hold a guy."[112]

The Emotional Cost of Sexually-Transmitted Diseases

As mentioned in the previous section, only half of the eight most prevalent sexually-transmitted diseases are curable. Since the suffering associated with non-curable STDs can last for a lifetime and can spread to partners or children, there is profound heartache when someone discovers they have such an infection. Those infected with HIV and other STDs are twice as likely to have depression and suffer from poor mental health than those without the disease. The National Institute of Mental Health claims HIV itself causes emotional, behavioral and other mental health problems.[113]

It is important to note that the emotional suffering associated with STDs can trigger further unrestrained sexual behaviors due to anxiety, which spreads the disease more. Of those who have been diagnosed with an STD, 25% do not tell their partners they have been infected.[114] Some individuals affected with an STD are so emotionally affected that they intentionally withhold the truth from their partner. This irresponsible behavior will make their partners experience the same suffering.[115] This furthers the spread of STDs, not only to their partner, but to future partners for both parties concerned. Laws vary from state to state within the United States, but for the most part it is illegal "to knowingly or recklessly transmit an STD." This means that all individuals who know they are infected with an STD have a moral and legal responsibility to tell every sexual partner that they are infected, or they could face a civil lawsuit, and in some states a criminal lawsuit.[116]

Having a sexually-transmitted disease is devastating. However, it is far worse to know that you have spread that disease to loved ones. The emotional harm caused by unrestrained sexual behaviors is life-long and pervasive. Spreading sexually-transmitted diseases to other people, merely for pleasure, is not love.

The Emotional Cost of Violence and Abuse

Post-traumatic stress disorder (PTSD) can develop after any traumatic incident. However, research shows that rape victims have more severe emotional and mental health concerns and are more likely to develop PTSD than others experiencing trauma.[117] In addition to PTSD, they experience depression, flash backs, and suicidal thoughts.

Victims of rape or sexual abuse often suffer from a negative self-identity. They start to see themselves as only sex-objects, having no inherent human value. Many also become gender-confused because of the sexual traumas they have experienced. They also lose their sense of safety and security. Victims of sexual violence and abuse can also suffer from disassociation, which is a "detachment from reality."[118] Sometimes they even come to blame themselves for the abuse they experienced. This can lead to self-harm. Victims "may use self-harm to cope with difficult or painful feelings."[119]

Tragically, countless children have been abused sexually. This can result in emotional trauma, which may haunt the children the rest of their lives. It should be obvious that the emotional consequences of the Sexual Holocaust transcend the physical consequences.

The Emotional Cost of Bondage and Slavery

Prostitutes and trafficked sex-workers experience much of the same emotional side-effects as those who have been raped: depression, flash backs, PTSD, and suicidal thoughts. Porn-stars, prostitutes, and victims of sex-trafficking also may have a false and negative self-identity and may start to view themselves as merely sex-objects. They too can suffer from disassociation and self-harm.

The Emotional Cost of Ubiquitous Abortion

Many women are finding that even though they may get a handle on the physical effects of an abortion, the emotional pain lasts throughout their life. The emotional pain caused by having an abortion varies from woman to woman, but includes regret, shame, and guilt. Abortions cause mental health issues such as insomnia, eating disorders, depression and suicidal thoughts. Many women acknowledge that having an abortion affected them more than they expected.[120]

A study published in 2017 by Priscilla K. Coleman, a professor at Bowling Green State University, showed that just under 32% of the participants who had recently had abortions, claimed there were no benefits to having an abortion.[121] The study also revealed that the benefits of having an abortion may not be as expected. Of those that did claim there had been a positive benefit, those benefits included: "spiritual growth, involvement in pro-life efforts, and reaching out to other women who were considering the procedure or had obtained an abortion."[122] However, the negatives expressed by the participants far out-weighed the positives and included: "deep feelings of loss, existential concerns, and declines in quality of life, feelings about termination of a life, regret, shame, guilt, depression, anxiety, compromised self-appraisals, and self-destructive behaviors."[123]

As we can see, unrestrained sexual behavior causes both physical and emotional harms that combine to increase total human suffering. However, the emotional pain is often much worse than the physical pain. It lasts longer and has a deeper effect. Even if we could remove all physical pain and suffering, there would still be profound emotional harm caused by unrestrained sexual behavior. People would still suffer from loneliness, rejection, depression, and suicide.

LONELINESS

The Internet, handheld devices, and artificial personalities are impacting the way humans communicate with each other. Historically, people have interacted face to face, but as technology has changed, so has our interaction. All human relationships are undergoing a tech-influenced change—even our sexual relationships.

An intimate and committed sexual relationship with a special loved one can be a great joy. However, with the influence of technology, people are increasingly seeking sexual experiences through virtual reality, screens, or social media. People are settling for degrading experiences because they do not have real, intimate relationships with one another. This type of behavior gives a momentary high (like a drug) but then leads to loneliness. This happens because these types of experiences are superficial. People withdraw from real relationships because virtual relations are easy and involve no emotional commitment. As the experiences increase in frequency and intensity, it becomes an addiction, and loneliness and shame are amplified.

According to Dr. Stephanie Cacioppo, director of the Brain Dynamics Lab at the University of Chicago, "loneliness is a state of mind characterized by a dissociation between what an individual wants or expects from a relationship and what that individual experiences in that relationship."[124] Dr. Cacioppo makes the point that because loneliness is a state of mind, one does not have to be physically alone to be lonely. This means that even though someone may not have physically withdrawn from relationships, they can still experience loneliness.

The dramatic increase in loneliness over the past few decades is primarily due to the ideas promoted through the sexual revolution. The sexual revolution is helping to drive the increase of loneliness through hardcore entertainment (pornography), softcore entertainment (television and movies), and social media. Hardcore pornography physically leads to loneliness because of its addictive nature (as discussed in the section above). It also leads to emotional loneliness because it replaces real people with images. Hardcore pornography draws people away from one another, out of the world of reality and into the lonely world of fantasy. It creates a dissociation between sexual expectations and actual sexual experiences, increasing a sense of loneliness. Lonely individuals look to pornography and personal physical release as a substitute for real relationships. This leads to further isolation and loneliness, which becomes a vicious cycle. This cycle has an accumulative effect, increasing both addiction and loneliness. Most pornography users try to hide their addiction, causing even deeper loneliness and, therefore, more isolation and a stronger feeling of the need for pornography.

Naomi Wolf, captures the pervasive sense of loneliness caused by pornography, when she writes this about our college campuses today:

"The young women who talk to me on campuses about the effect of pornography on their intimate lives speak of feeling that they can never measure up, that they can never ask for what they want; and that if they do not offer what porn offers, they cannot expect to hold a guy. The young men talk about what it is like to grow up learning about sex from porn, and how it is not helpful to them in trying to figure out how to be with a real woman. Mostly, when I ask about loneliness, a deep, sad silence descends on audiences of young men and young women alike. They know they are lonely together, even when conjoined, and that this imagery is a big part of that loneliness."[125]

The effect of softcore entertainment may not be as obvious, but it has the same basic effect. Most humans in this culture spend more time interacting with phones, iPads, or other technology than they do interacting with other human beings. Movies and television encourage certain expectations regarding sex and relationships—expectations that are unrealistic. For example, the media consistently indicates that every lead character needs to be widely-admired, sexy, and sexually active. As we just mentioned, having expectations that are not met by the relationships in one's real life causes loneliness and the turn to fantasy. Softcore entertainment has become the modern sex-education teacher, but it is normalizing harmful versions of sexuality by promoting examples of shallow, broken, unhealthy, and degrading sexual relationships. All this deepens the loneliness that is now being experienced by more than half of all Americans. Like all modern media, softcore entertainment appeals to people's fantasies. Therefore, the entertainment media today strives to "hook" their audience using a mix of sex, violence, and shock value.

Social media is exacerbating this situation. Social media perpetuates the false concept that people are genuinely connecting through these social platforms. In reality, it is simply amplifying loneliness by replacing a person with a screen. Face-to-face communication has been replaced by an email, text, or instant message. Handshakes, hugs, and other forms of healthy physical touch or displays of emotions have been replaced with emoji's. People have always felt an innate desire to belong; however, now social media keeps us up-to-date on what everyone is doing. This "snap-shot" into everyone's life is causing individuals to suffer extreme forms of fear that they are "missing out." This is commonly known as FOMO, the "fear of missing out." Because our example for healthy relationships has been distorted by hardcore entertainment, softcore entertainment, and social media, we no longer know how to have genuine, intimate relationships and, therefore, we silently suffer loneliness—even while surrounded by people, entertainment, and technology.

Loneliness may seem like a minor concern, but if it is persistent and acute, it can be emotionally devastating. According to Dr. Vivek H. Murthy, former Surgeon General of the United States, "loneliness and weak social connections are associated with a reduction in lifespan similar to that caused by smoking 15 cigarettes a day and even greater than that associated with obesity."[126] Loneliness triggers hormones in our body, which affect our immune system and leave us susceptible to infections and other diseases, like cancer, cardiovascular disease, and diabetes.[127]

Unlike the physical harms of the Sexual Holocaust, loneliness is hard to quantify. However, there are studies that show that loneliness is now an epidemic. Loneliness is one of the top fears in the world.[128] Over the past 50 years, the rates of loneliness have doubled.[129] In the United States nearly half the population admits to feeling lonely, left out, and isolated.[130] Only about half the American population has in-person, meaningful, daily interactions with friends or family.[131] It is not just the young (isolated because of their screens) or the old (isolated because of their health), who suffer from loneliness. Research shows that people can suffer from loneliness in all stages of their life. A study conducted across one university campus, showed that participants "who engaged in penetrative sex hookups subsequently reported an increase in both depressive symptoms and feelings of loneliness."[132]

It is striking to see that the sexual revolution promised intimacy and fulfillment through sexual relationships, but the real consequence has been an increase in loneliness and a decline in meaningful relationships. Loneliness is the least of the emotional harms of the Sexual Holocaust, yet health specialists say it is a epidemic. As we will see, the following emotional harms are even more destructive.

REJECTION

Rejection is the spurning of another person's affections. It is not a new concept; however, the Sexual Holocaust is amplifying rejection. Rejection directly impacts our sense of human worth by undermining our identity. A primary reason the Sexual Holocaust is so harmful is because it corrupts our sense of self. In this hyper-sexualized culture, an individual's worth is mostly measured by *cool* and *sexy*. In reality, we are all quite ordinary human beings. *Cool* is just a front and *sexy* is fleeting and largely fabricated. Media drives society by insisting that everyone must be cool and sexy. This is influencing people to desperately try to impress each other with fronts and fabrications. This is because they believe that if they are not cool or sexy they have no worth. This notion is totally wrong—human value vastly transcends cool and sexy—as will be discussed in the "Spiritual Section" of this overview.

The Sexual Holocaust corrupts people's identity by setting them up against porn-stars and people who have had surgical make-overs. In this hyper-sexualized environment, we are all tempted to measure our worth by our amount of sex-appeal. Countless lonely, normal people feel totally inadequate, in light of the new sexual norms. Men feel inadequate in personal relationships because they only know how to relate to images on a screen. They are generally not getting married because they do not know what real love is. Women are not getting married because so many men lust for visual images, rejecting normal woman as if they are worthless. Likewise, women who see themselves as cool or sexy, reject normal guys in the same way as men are rejecting women.

This widespread rejection, which is based upon hyper-sexualized standards, is best seen in the hookup culture. The hookup culture is perpetuating ubiquitous, mass rejection in universities and college campuses around the world. Dr. Lisa Wade analyzed the hookup culture in her book *American Hookup*. Through personal student testimonies and research across the nation, Dr. Wade says, "Using indicators like hotness, blondness, fraternity membership, and athletic prowess, students form a working consensus about who is hookup-worthy."[133] As one student put it, "I can't expect any of the girls I'll meet on a Friday night to care about my personality or my favorite books."[134] He complained that girls only slept with him for his good looks or to share his weed. He admitted that he acts distant or dismissive towards women to avoid being rejected himself. The testimonies gathered from students across the United States shows that the Sexual Holocaust changes our human identity by making us into sex-objects for one another. In the hookup culture, people tend to use others to gain social status, drugs, etc. The people who are used are rejected once the user gets what they want, or if the individual can no longer provide these things.

According to Dr. Wade, the hookup culture also perpetuates rejection because students need a way to justify their promiscuity. In her book, *American Hookup*, she explains how students go through an almost ritualistic mating ceremony to choose who to hook-up with for the night. However, in the morning, they somehow have to justify their actions. They do this by (1) using alcohol as an excuse, (they claim that when you are drunk you cannot be responsible for your actions) or (2) immediately rejecting whoever they just hooked-up with. If they were initially friends they are demoted to associates, if associates, strangers, and if strangers, they won't acknowledge each other's existence.

The hurt caused by rejection surpasses the physical harms discussed earlier and even surpasses the hurt of loneliness. According to a functional magnetic resonance imaging (FMRI) study, our brain reacts the same way to rejection as it does to physical pain. This means we can experience the same intensity of pain when we experience rejection as we do with physical pain.[135] Not only is the pain from rejection just as intense as physical pain, the pain is more vivid and longer-lasting. According to Dr. Guy Winch, a licensed psychologist, rejection hurts more than any physical pain because, as humans, we relive social pain more vividly than physical pain. If we recall a time when we were physically hurt, it does not normally make our body start hurting again. However, if we recall a time when we were rejected, we hurt all over again.[136] Dr. Winch suggests that even recalling a time in our lives when we were rejected can significantly lower our IQ, hurt our short-term memory, and harm our decision making.[137] "Social rejection increases anger, anxiety, depression, jealousy and sadness. It reduces performance on difficult intellectual tasks, and can also contribute to aggression and poor impulse control," says Dr. C. Nathan DeWall, a psychologist at the University of Kentucky.[138] "In 2001, the Surgeon General of the U.S. issued a report stating that rejection was a greater risk for adolescent violence than drugs, poverty, or gang membership."[139]

Rejection is seen on all levels, in many different areas of life. However, the Sexual Holocaust, the hookup culture, and the media are causing unprecedented harm by profoundly undermining our identity, humanity, and self-worth. The sexual revolution has made us consumers of one another, but this is not our true identity. This cannot give us lasting human worth.

DEPRESSION

The *National Institute for Mental Health* defines depression (clinical depression) as "a mood disorder that causes distressing symptoms that affect how you feel, think, and handle daily activities."[140] There are several types of depression, which include: major depression, persistent depressive disorder (dysthymia), perinatal depression, seasonal affective disorder, and psychotic depression. Depression can be caused by a number of factors. Most people believe that depression is caused by an imbalance of chemicals in your body. This can be one cause; however, "researchers believe that—more important than levels of specific brain chemicals—nerve cell connections, nerve cell growth, and the functioning of nerve circuits have a major impact on depression."[141] Genes can also impact depression. Our genes turn on and off throughout our life, and this effects our emotional health.[142] However, studies may be suggesting that these biological factors can be due more to our lifestyle and environment than previously thought.

According to Dr. Rashmi Nemade:

"Many people with major depressive disorder report that a stressful event caused their first or second depressive episode. Research suggests that later depressive episodes (starting with the third) tend to develop in the absence of any particular stressor. Some scientists call this phenomenon the 'kindling effect,' or 'kindling-sensitization hypothesis.' According to this idea, initial depressive episodes create changes in the brain's chemistry that make it more likely that future episodes of depression will develop (or kindle, if you think about a spark starting a fire). Since early episodes of depression make a person more sensitive to developing later episodes, even a small series of daily hassles can trigger ongoing depressive episodes."[143]

The *German LAC Depression Study* showed that more than 75% of those suffering from depression experienced some form of trauma as a child.[144] This study also showed that multiple traumatic experiences lead to more severe symptoms of depression. It also suggested that children who suffered from emotional or sexual abuse exhibited more severe symptoms of depression as an adult. "Epigenetic studies further substantiate the finding that a genetic vulnerability will only lead to depression if the individual experienced simultaneous early traumatization."[145] It is, therefore, not difficult to see that though depression may be triggered by biological causes, there is an underlying cause of trauma that initiates a significant portion of depression cases.

Depression impacts the global community. According to the WHO, "300 million people around the world have depression."[146] Depression is the third leading disease worldwide and the first leading disease in middle- and high-income countries.[147] According to *The Blue Cross Blue Shield* data report for 2016, depression in America has risen by 33 percent since 2013.[148] Depending on the age group, the percentage of those suffering from depression has increased as much as 63%. Psychologists debate what has caused this increase, but some suggest social media, substance abuse, isolation, trauma, debt, etc. Most of these causes of depression can be linked, directly or indirectly, to the Sexual Holocaust.

In the previous section, we looked at how unrestrained sexual behavior causes physical pain and trauma. It is clear to see that such behaviors lead to depression. Even after a traumatic experience, people may suffer life-long depression because of the way life experiences change one's brain. Again, the emotional harms of the Sexual Holocaust out-weigh the physical harms.

SUICIDE

In high-income communities, research has shown that suicide is directly linked to depression and alcohol use.[149] However, suicide is also linked with "moments of crisis with a breakdown in the ability to deal with life stresses, such as financial problems, relationship break-up or chronic pain and illness."[150]

"In addition, experiencing conflict, disaster, violence, abuse, or loss and a sense of isolation are strongly associated with suicidal behavior. Suicide rates are also high amongst vulnerable groups who experience discrimination, such as refugees and migrants; indigenous peoples; lesbian, gay, bisexual, transgender, intersex (LGBTI) persons; and prisoners."[151]

Suicide rates are increasing, and the concern is global. According to the WHO, 800,000 people a year commit suicide, about 1 person every 40 seconds.[152] "There are indications that for each adult who died by suicide there may have been more than 20 others attempting suicide."[153] Suicide "is the second leading cause of death among 15-29 year-olds, globally."[154]

Suicide is the consequence of a major emotional breakdown in one's life. It is a consequence of traumas or stresses that seem too large to handle. The Sexual Holocaust is responsible for causing vast amounts of pain, trauma, and emotional suffering, which are the primary causes of suicide. Unrestrained sexual behavior is a leading factor in suicide. In the next section, we will see how unrestrained sexual behavior is wreaking havoc on our society.

EMOTIONAL HARM SUMMARY

The Sexual Holocaust has caused horrendous physical harm and even deeper and longer-lasting emotional harm. We have seen in multiple instances that unrestrained sexual behavior causes physical and emotional pain. People often respond to such pain by using further unrestrained sexual behaviors as an escape mechanism. This perpetuates the vicious cycle that is fueling the Sexual Holocaust. In the next section, we will zoom out still further, widening our view as we look at the social harms of the Sexual Holocaust.

CHAPTER 3

HARMFUL SOCIAL CONSEQUENCES OF THE SEXUAL HOLOCAUST

Healthy societies prosper when there are stable social institutions in place. These institutions, such as marriage, family, schools, and political systems, help define society, give it structure, and help bring purpose to life. Societies change as the culture changes, as technology changes, and as new discoveries bring change. Change can be good. However, the change brought about by the sexual revolution seems to have primarily resulted in the destabilization of society.

In this chapter we will look at four social consequences of the Sexual Holocaust: (1) The breakdown of marriage, (2) The breakdown of the family, (3) The redefining of "child," and (4) Institutionalizing "anything-goes" sexuality.

We will see how these social harms amplify and transcend the physical and emotional pain discussed in the previous two sections.

THE BREAKDOWN OF MARRIAGE

As the sexual revolution has spread and gained momentum, traditional institutions, like marriage, have been systematically weakened. This began with the idea of "free love." Ever since that time, marriage rates have been declining rapidly. Currently, only 50% of Americans are getting married in the United States.[155] In the 1960s the marriage rate was 72% of Americans.[156] This rapid decline in marriage is not unique to the United States—it is a global trend. In Europe, only 4.3 people per every 1,000 inhabitants get married.[157] According to a census in 2018, the number of marriages recorded in South Korea were at the lowest they have been in recorded history.[158]

What is the driving force that is breaking down marriage? The answer is deep and complex because many things are working together to undermine marriage. In this section, we will discuss a few major factors that have led to the breakdown of marriage. As mentioned already, unrestrained sexual behaviors, like hookups and pornography, lead to the breakdown of marriage. Other concerns, such as economic instability and population decline, may also slow marriage rates.

The breakdown of marriage is not just due to fewer marriages. It is also due to higher rates of divorce. No-fault divorce, where a spouse can get out of the commitment at any time, breaks apart the family and makes the marriage commitment minimal. As of 2017, in India, marriage rates have remained high, but divorce rates have doubled in the past two decades.[159] In the United States, the divorce rates have decreased recently; however, this is simply because so many people are not getting married any more.

Cohabitation is another factor contributing to the breakdown of marriage. It is increasing while marriage is in decline. This means that when people break-up from cohabitating, it is not recorded as a divorce.[160] The revolving door of relationships is not slowing down, it is picking up speed. The increase in cohabitation simply means that people do not want to be committed to each other.

The redefinition of marriage is also contributing to the breakdown of marriage. In 2015 in the United States, the Supreme Court declared that the 14th amendment "requires a state to license a marriage between two people of the same sex."[161] Since that time, advocacy for "anything-goes" sexuality has exploded. "Marriage" is now largely whatever people want it to be. The term is losing its meaning.

When marriage becomes casual, arbitrary, or ambiguous, it sets the stage for "anything-goes" households where people can come and go on a whim. If marriage is "whatever arrangement is preferred," then logically, we can expect weekend marriages, polygamous marriages, incestuous marriages, child marriages, and perhaps even bestial marriages. This may sound extreme, but not in the context of the rapid social breakdown we are witnessing. Currently, polyamorous relationships are not yet legalized in all fifty states, but are already common. They are already legal in Utah, as long as couples do not require multiple marriage licenses.[162] Adult incest is not a criminal act in Rhode Island nor New Jersey.[163] Currently, the minimal age of marriage varies from state to state[164] and is clearly subject to change. In many Muslim nations, children as young as nine are given in marriage. As of 2017, Hawaii, Kentucky, New Mexico, West Virginia and Wyoming do not have laws against sexual conduct with animals.[165]

Once society says marriage is arbitrary and love is relative, *everything* becomes permissible—including intimate, emotional and physical relationships with non-humans. We mentioned bestiality above; however, technology has paved the way for a new type of relationship that is replacing not only marriage, but human-to-human physical relationships. A technology, similar to the Google or Alexa artificial personalities, has been created by the Japanese company, Gatebox, which advertises a new breed of "partner." It "is designed to replace a real-life relationship with a virtual girlfriend." Pre-orders became available in December of 2016.[166]

However, marriage is not just being replaced by artificial, *digital* relationships. Technology is making a way for artificial, *physical* relationships by taking "sex toys" to a whole new level. Sex toys and sex dolls are already commonly marketed around the globe, but extremely realistic robots are beginning to replace, not the toys, but human partners. Dr. Ian Pearson, a futurist and speaker in London, UK, predicts that "people will be having both emotional and casual sex with robots by 2030." He also predicts that "human-robot sex will eventually overtake human-human sex by 2050."[167] This may seem shocking; however, Dr. Pearson believes that, "like porn, once a lot of people use it [robots] and it becomes normalized, people won't be freaked out by it anymore."[168]

> "A lot of people will still have reservations about sex with robots at first but gradually as they get used to them, as the AI and mechanical behavior and their feel improves, and they *start to become friends* with strong emotional bonds, that squeamishness will gradually evaporate."[169]

Pornography, as we have already discussed, has conditioned our society to accept that real, live men and women are often not as appealing as what is seen on a screen. Technology is now offering something visually and physically appealing that in some ways will transcend human-to-human sex. A robot can look like anyone (or anything) you want. This new emotional and sexual friendship with an artificial being may begin to replace not only marriages, but human intimacy. Will the Supreme Court eventually say the 14th Amendment must be applied to human-AI relationships?

"Anything-goes" sexuality is rapidly transforming marriage into any mutually acceptable and convenient arrangement. This is a long way from the time-proven and stabilizing-institution of marriage of the past. This type of unrestrained sexuality is amplifying human suffering. As we will see in the following sections, once marriage breaks down within a country, the country itself will break down. Once we define marriage as "whatever," the definition of *family* becomes highly arbitrary as does the definition of *child/parent*. Without stable marriages and families, people have no close network of support and no model of real relationships. As we will see in the next section, the breakdown of marriage is causing social harm that is global and will have unforeseen consequences that are hard to imagine.

THE BREAKDOWN OF FAMILY

As marriage has become marginalized in society, so has *family*. Today, families are in decline, they are increasingly "fluid." Families are being formed and reformed according to human convenience, rather than naturally formed bonds that result from marriage. Fewer and fewer children grow up in an intact, stable family. Fewer and fewer children have a meaningful "father."

The Loss of Family and the Decline of Nations

As marriage rates decline, so do birth rates. Japan, for example, saw its biggest population decline in 2018. The Japanese birth rate is amazingly low and continues to drop, while death rates continue to rise. More than 20% of the population is over 65.[170] Irregular, unstable employment[171] may be one reason that young Japanese men and women give for not getting married. However, there is a much more pervasive reason—unrestrained sexual behavior. Marriage is being undermined by pornography, and real relationships are being replaced by "a new breed of partner." Japan, though just a small island, is the 4th leading nation to visit the website Pornhub.[172] In fact, "hentai," which is short for the Japanese term *hentai seiyoku*, is one of the most searched for words in pornography searches. It means "perverse sexual desire" and is used to broadly describe Japan's genre of anime pornography. However, pornography is not the only harm that is impacting the Japanese culture and leading to the loss of family. As mentioned above, the Japanese company Gatebox has offered an alternative type of relationship—digital relationships. Technology is truly replacing the family. Marriage and birth rates have declined so much that Japan's population size is imploding.

Japan is not the only nation that is being affected by the breakdown of marriage. In South Korea, on average, women are having 0.98 children in their lifetime (2.1

children per woman is required to maintain population size).[173] Without marriage, without family, without sufficient children, these nations will implode in just a few decades. Lack of children means a population of senior citizens and eventual economic collapse.

Divorce

Divorce is devastating families. As children watch their parents "fall out of love" with one another, they learn some difficult lessons about life. They learn that relationships are not stable and are subject to radical change. They learn that sexual or romantic love is not lasting and is basically arbitrary, subject to emotional whims. They learn to live without a mother's or father's daily and direct influence. The instability that divorce creates within a family leaves children emotionally compromised.

In the *Journal of the American Academy of Child & Adolescent Psychiatry* a study shows that "significant numbers of children suffer for many years from psychological and social difficulties" associated with divorce. Children of divorced families "experience heightened anxiety in forming enduring attachments" later in life.[174] Children of different ages respond differently to divorce. For the younger child, the child's world is a dependent one, closely connected to parents who are favored companions. Young children are heavily reliant on parental care, with the family as the major locus of their life. However, divorce destroys the child's trust in their parents, as suddenly life is filled with instability. For older children, "the adolescent world is a more independent one, more separated and distant from parents, more self-sufficient, where friends have become favored companions, and where the major locus of one's social life now extends outside of the family and into a larger world of life experience."[175] This often leads the older children to have anger towards their parents. An older child will often "disregard family discipline and take care of himself since parents have failed to keep the commitments to the family that were originally made."[176]

With divorce, a once stable environment becomes filled with uncertainty. Children wonder if parents will stop loving them, as they stopped loving each other. They wonder if they will lose both parents as they have already lost one. Regardless of the age of the child, divorce brings negative changes to what family looks like.

Cohabitation and Promiscuity

Cohabitation has largely replaced marriage, and it is becoming the new normal in terms of what "family" means. "So much so," says Wendy D. Manning, Distinguished Research Professor, "that by age 12, 40 percent of American children will have spent at least part of their lives in a cohabiting household."[177]

As of 2016, 66% of married couples cohabited before they got married. In the past 25 years, cohabitation has doubled in frequency among middle-aged and younger Americans. Manning notes that several factors decrease a child's well-being when living in a cohabitating family. These include: poverty, reduced education, and absence of legal protections associated with parental marriage. Dr. Manning says that the most detrimental factor to a child's health when living in a cohabiting family is the instability of the family unit. These children see their "parents" break up more often than married couples, which leads to further instability in the children's lives, including instability in their own relationships. Although cohabiting families with two committed, biological parents appears to "offer many of the same health, cognitive, and behavioral benefits that stable married biological parent families provide," Manning says that "children who are born to cohabiting parents appear to experience enduring deficits of psychosocial wellbeing."[178]

Furthermore, cohabitation often means little or no sexual fidelity. Children in cohabiting families are more likely to have to navigate complex relationships where sexual partners come and go, with the current "father" often not being the biological father. A child may experience numerous "daddies" who may not act like a daddy at all. In polyamorous situations the child becomes even more disoriented by the various "parents" and "relatives." Likewise, as more parents come and go, so do their children, making the term 'brother' or 'sister' increasingly ambiguous. In such cases, non-biological "siblings" will tend to have only superficial relationships—like roommates. Likewise, "grandparents," "aunts," and "uncles" may simply be temporary housemates. In the context of families where the adults are promiscuous, the various children and adults do not really see each other as family. Under these circumstances sexual relations can be fluid, and may be in some way incestuous (regardless of biological relatedness). The children may not feel safe even when at home. This type of familial chaos can be especially destructive because children desire to develop their identity around a trusted role model, but such a role model may be transient or absent entirely.

It is often claimed that economics and income have more to do with family stability than marriage itself. However, according to studies done by the *Institute for Family Studies*, "in the overwhelming majority of countries, the most educated cohabiting parents still have a far higher rate of break-up than the lowest educated married couples." They "showed that children have more stable family lives when born within marriage regardless of their mother's educational background."[179]

Reproductive Technology and Selective Abortions

Today, reproductive technologies are radically transforming what "normal family" looks like. The gender of a developing embryo can now easily be determined genetically. Indeed, many other genetic traits can likewise be determined. In China, India, and ten other nations, such genetic traits are being screened out by using selective abortions. For example, "differential gender mortality has been a documented problem for decades and led to reports in the early 1990s of 100 million 'missing women' across the developing world."[180] Though the practice of abandoning unwanted babies to die is not new, technology is now assisting with this process by terminating them *in utero*. These types of selective abortions began to be available in about 1985.

Selective abortions are happening on such a large scale in China and India that many more male babies are born than are female babies, resulting in a shortage of girls and women. "The resulting large cohorts of 'surplus' young men are only now reaching reproductive age."[181] This large number of men are now single because they have little prospect of finding a stable female companion. An article in the journal *Proceedings of the National Academy of Sciences* (PNAS), says that "in many communities today there are growing numbers of young men in the lower echelons of society who are marginalized because of lack of family prospects and who have little outlet for sexual energy."[182] The article suggests that this "surplus' of males" is leading to "antisocial behavior and violence, threatening societal stability and security."[183] Because this large number of men have sexual needs that are not being met by the small population of women, the sex industry is expanding in these nations and in many ways, expanding to include "more unacceptable practices like coercion and trafficking."[184] Besides the sex market, violence, and homicides are also on the increase. "It is a consistent finding across cultures that an overwhelming percentage of violent crime is perpetrated by young, unmarried, low-status males."[185] A study in India concluded that there is "a clear link between sex ratio and violence as a whole, not just violence against women as might be assumed when there is a shortage of females."[186] This type of mounting violence is a global concern, as the PNAS article explains:

"These men are likely to be attracted to military-type organizations, with the potential to be a trigger for large-scale domestic and international violence. With 40% of the world's population living in China and India...the sex imbalance could impact regional and global security, especially because the surrounding countries of Pakistan, Taiwan, Nepal, and Bangladesh also have high sex ratios."[187]

Though there are laws that discourage selective abortion, these laws are hard to enforce. In the United States, only "9 states ban abortions for reason of sex selection."[188] These types of laws are often opposed by those claiming to advocate women's rights. People want to promote a women's right to choose what to do with her womb; however, by allowing selective abortions, families and nations are imploding and global violence is increasing.

The issue does not just end with gender selection. *In utero* babies can be screened for any genetic trait and then aborted as desired. In the United States, it is reported that only "2 states prohibit abortions for reasons of race."[189] As our world continues to become more hyper-sexualized, babies can be screened for traits that will make them more appealing. As society tries to control what our children should look like, our world moves further and further into confusion and chaos.

Surrogacy

Surrogacy is another type of reproductive procedure that is circumventing what normal "family" looks like. There are two types of surrogacy: (1) traditional surrogacy, where the surrogate mother becomes pregnant through artificial insemination and, therefore, has a genetic connection with the child born for the intended parents, or (2) gestational surrogacy, where an egg is surgically removed from a woman of choice and fertilized by the sperm of a man of choice in a test tube (*in vitro fertilization*). The fertilized egg can then be implanted in a different woman, the gestational carrier. Neither the sperm donor, nor the egg donor, nor the gestational carrier need be a legal parent. The people who "own" the resulting child can be anyone who can pay for it.

The birth of a surrogate child can involve up to five adult participants—the surrogate, the sperm donor, the egg donor, and the two prospective "parents" who will legally own the baby. Surrogacy can be complicated for all parties, but can be especially difficult for the surrogate and the baby. The *Iranian Journal of Reproductive Medicine* revealed in 2014 that "surrogate moms experience significant emotional attachment to the children they carry...Researchers concluded, 'surrogacy pregnancy should be considered as a high-risk emotional experience because many surrogate mothers may face negative experiences.'"[190] According to the *British Journal of Medicine*, besides the emotional risks, surrogate mothers also suffer from: risk of Caesarian sections, longer hospital stays, gestational diabetes, fetal growth restriction, pre-eclampsia, and premature birth. Many surrogates are diagnosed with post-traumatic stress disorder (PTSD) after their delivery.

In a perfect world, surrogacy seems like a good way to help stable couples who cannot have their own children. However, we do not live in a perfect world. Too often, people use each other. A surrogate mother is a woman who rents out her womb for the purpose of carrying and birthing a child for the benefit of another person (or couple). She has legal obligations to the people paying her. However, she is taking a serious risk in terms of medical complications and must endure all the hardships and pain associated with pregnancy and the emotional cost of giving up the baby she has carried and birthed. She even faces the remote possibility of death associated with complications. Surrogate mothers often face unjustified accusations from the intended parents in cases where unexpected health issues arise affecting the baby or if the intended parents have to pay for medical complications. Jennifer Lahl, at the Center for Bioethics and Culture Network, sums up surrogacy this way: "surrogacy is another form of the commodification of women's bodies...and degrades a pregnancy to a service and a baby to a product."[191]

Surrogacy does not just affect surrogate mothers. It has an effect on the surrogate children. The University of Cambridge published a study in *Journal of Child Psychology and Psychiatry* that suggested that surrogate children struggle with increased emotional risks, such as depression around the age of 7, as they try to understand what it means to have been a surrogate child. Studies have shown that the lack of a gestational connection with their mothers is more detrimental to a child then not having a genetic connection with either parent. This shows that there is a physical, emotional, social, and arguably a spiritual connection that forms between a child and the birth mother. Even though a surrogate child raised in a stable family unit can overcome this, it is not without its challenges. The *American Society for Reproductive Medicine* says, that while it is a parent's choice whether to disclose the origins of their child's birth, the *Society* strongly encourages disclosure because of the instability that is created as a child reaches their adolescence and works on forming their own identity.[192] The question of whether surrogate parents should tell their children becomes more complicated with homosexual couples, because procreation requires male and female gametes. Children of homosexual couples will quickly understand that their parents could not possibly be their biological parents—even if those parents do not disclose to the child their surrogate birth.

Surrogacy is creating instability on many levels. It is increasing class division in our society. Surrogacy is an expensive process, costing anywhere between $90,000 and $130,000.[193] This is only widening the gap between the wealthy and poor. Surrogacy is only available to those who can afford it. Surrogate compensation can be $50,000 to $80,000 depending on experience, insurance, location, and other factors. The substantial pay to surrogate mothers is very attractive to women who are struggling financially. They can still work another job while carrying someone else's baby. However, as seen above, being a surrogate is not easy and can leave the surrogate with piles of medical bills and serious medical and emotional problems. The "mother" who will "own" the new baby does not have to get stretch marks, or gain weight, or spoil her figure, or even give birth. This will surely widen the gap between the haves and the have-nots.

Surrogacy is still being debated within the United States, where success rates among fertility clinics are the best in the world.[194] Surrogacy in some parts of the world is much riskier and can be much more demeaning for the surrogate mother. Surrogacy is not legal in all states, nor are all states surrogacy-friendly. This ongoing debate should give us pause to consider the long-term effects of surrogacy on family and society.

The effect of surrogacy on family is an important issue; however, it is not the only issue to consider. As our technology and medical capabilities advance, we are learning new ways to make designer babies by editing the genetic code. Surrogacy and *in vitro* fertilization have thrown open the door for human cloning and human gene editing. The first genetically engineered babies have already been born. As we will see in the following section, once the definition of marriage changes, so does the family, and so does the child. Sadly, children are becoming commodities.

REDEFINING THE "CHILD"

Altering the definition of marriage has led to a new type of family and both of these developments are leading to a new type of child. It starts simply enough, with surrogacy—giving the intended parents the choice of who will be the surrogate mother and who will be the genetic donors for their children. With advancements in genetic research, parents will be able to pay to have their child genetically engineered. This will let people *choose* their child's genetic make-up, right down to eye color. It is profoundly ironic since in western culture we obsess over keeping everything "natural" and largely shun any type of GMO food, yet we are rapidly moving toward Frankenstein-type experiments with our children and have already started making GMO babies.

As of 2018, "the *Nuffield Council on Bioethics* has concluded that editing the DNA of a human embryo, sperm, or egg to influence the characteristics of a future person ('heritable genome editing') *could be morally permissible.*"

"The Council recommends that two overarching principles should guide the use of 'heritable genome editing interventions' for them to be *ethically acceptable*: (1) they must be intended to secure, and be consistent with, the welfare of the future person; and (2) they should not increase disadvantage, discrimination or division in society."[195]

It is still currently illegal to conduct "heritable genome editing" in the United Kingdom. However, the debate is ongoing, and the relevant research is being pushed forward rapidly.

Even though experiments have shown that DNA alterations can reduce the risk of some diseases, "scientists at the Wellcome Sanger Institute have discovered that CRISPR/Cas9 gene editing can cause greater genetic damage in cells than was previously thought."[196] The journal *Nature Biotechnology* reported in July 2018 that "standard tests for detecting DNA changes miss[ed] finding this genetic damage."[197]

Genetic modification is illegal in most parts of the world; however, Dr. He Jiankui of the Southern University of Science and Technology in Shenzhen, China, "says he used human embryos modified with the gene-editing technique CRISPR to create twin girls."[198] These girls are literally genetically modified organisms (GMOs). He modified their genetic code to reduce their risk of contracting HIV, since their father was HIV positive. Jiankui is currently facing an investigation and has been put on unpaid leave by the Southern University of Science and Technology.

Human cloning is the next logical step in designer babies. Cloning, like genome editing, creates new physical, emotional, and social harms that we can not yet imagine.

"In 2002 the National Academy of Sciences released a report calling for a legal ban on human cloning. The report concluded that the high rate of health problems in cloned animals suggests that such an effort in humans would be highly dangerous for the mother and developing embryo and is likely to fail. Beyond safety, the possibility of cloning humans also raises a variety of social issues like the psychological issues that would result for a cloned child who is the identical twin of his or her parent."[199]

What were once simple childhood problems (scrapes on knees, school bullies, and becoming your own little person) are not simple anymore. Children are now being hyper-sexualized. They are now sex-objects, commodities, and experimental animals. The sexual revolution is changing the face of childhood. We are already making and selling babies—so why not designer babies? Why can't we grow biologically enhanced babies for sex appeal—or for war? Will genetically modified humans be sub-human? Super-human? Will they be human at all? Who will decide?

The next generation of children will have to wrestle with more and more complex personal dilemmas regarding their identity. Who are their *real* parents? Are they clones? In a world determined to have sexual liberation at any cost, we will have to reexamine what it means to be human. We have already seen how the Sexual Holocaust is redefining basic institutions like marriage and family. We can only wonder how much instability and chaos will follow this breakdown before responsible individuals say enough is enough. In the following section, we will discuss another major factor that is amplifying the social harm resulting from the Sexual Holocaust. We will see how all of this confusion, instability, and harm is being aggressively promoted through our most powerful social institutions.

Institutionalizing "Anything-Goes" Sexuality

Throughout this overview, we have been trying to grasp the full scope of the Sexual Holocaust. Our hope is that responsible individuals will start to understand the magnitude of the current crisis and will help reverse the direction of where things are going. However, this will be difficult because most of the major social institutions of our day are aggressively promoting "anything-goes" sexuality.

Humans are born with a basic sexual drive, but how that sex drive is manifested is largely affected by *learned behavior*. Our sexuality is greatly influenced by what we *see*, what we *are exposed to,* and what we *choose*. Our basic sexual drive can be easily high-jacked and misdirected by various *learned behaviors*. Many extremely destructive learned behaviors are now being taught through the media and throughout the culture. We cannot presume these types of learned behaviors are necessarily natural or inborn. Many behaviors are being *promoted, modeled,* and *cultivated*. Early exposures to unnatural or extreme forms of sexual stimulation can result in lifelong struggles.

Unrestrained sexuality has always been a problem; however, now it is being wholeheartedly endorsed and promoted by the institutions we have traditionally trusted. This includes the media, the government, the education system, and many religious institutions. We will discuss a few of these.

The Media

We will start with the entertainment industry. We have emphasized that the hyper-sexualization of our culture has been primarily driven through the sex-saturated entertainment industry. Great harm is caused when sexuality is institutionalized through hardcore entertainment (pornography), softcore entertainment (movies and television), and social media. The entertainment industry now sets the standard or norm for sexual behavior. As mentioned earlier, hardcore entertainment is distributed and normalized by respected main-stream corporate giants of the entertainment industry and now accounts for a large part of all internet traffic. Hardcore entertainment is now promoted and easily accessible to everyone, including young children. Softcore entertainment has become the modern sex-education teacher, but it is normalizing harmful versions of sexuality by promoting examples of shallow, broken, unhealthy, and degrading sexual relationships. Social media has become a marketplace for sex. YouTube videos on the Kids Channel teach children how to pick up girls on Facebook (along with the myriad of swearing and sexual innuendos heard on these types of videos). Through everyday interaction with the entertainment industry, we are being trained to embrace unrestrained, liberated, "anything-goes" sexuality. This is clearly creating confusion in our individual lives and in our society. People view each other more and more as sex-objects, with women and young girls being the primary targets for objectification. However, it is not just the entertainment industry that is taking us down this road.

The Government

Government and radical political advocacy groups are also helping to promote and normalize "anything-goes" sexuality. Those who are using the government to push "anything-goes" sexuality are forcing their agenda on an unsuspecting population. A large fraction of the population is generally unaware of what is happening, or are deeply concerned about what is happening, but feel they are not free to express their concerns. Media and government have locked arms in their advocacy for "anything-goes" sexuality. They are no longer looking out for the wellbeing of the society.

Today, "rights" seems to be at odds with "responsibilities." In the western world, all kinds of "rights" are being demanded, with no regard for "responsibilities." Responsible governments should not promote unrestrained sexuality but should promote sexual responsibility. This is best for the individual and for society.

The Education System

Even within our state-run education systems, children are being taught from a young age they must embrace and endorse "anything-goes" sexuality or be shunned and labeled a hater or bigot. Our education systems are creating a standard for sexuality that is sexually explicit and extreme. This past May 2019, "the California Department of Education approved controversial changes to the state's health and sex education curriculum."[200] One book on the list of resources for parents, geared towards kindergarteners through third graders, shows cartoon pictures of male and female genitals and explains various types of sexuality. Through the educational system, 5 to 9-year-old children are being taught, in detail, extremely diverse (obscene) forms of sexual behavior. This means that well before a child's body is ready for sex, schools are *explicitly* teaching them how to engage in sex and are implicitly encouraging pre-puberty sexual experimentation.

Because of the hyper-sexualization of our culture, sex education is extremely important for children. However, children are not being adequately warned about the tragic consequences of unrestrained sexual behaviors. Instead, they are being taught how to celebrate and engage in unrestrained sexual behaviors at the earliest possible age. It appears that few schools are giving appropriate warnings and most schools are encouraging early experimentation and indulgence. This includes encouraging little children to toy with bisexual behaviors, play with cross-dressing, and fantasize radical gender transformations. In light of the Sexual Holocaust, this public education direction is destructive on a level that is almost beyond description. Encouraging early and unbounded sexual experimentation will lead many children into identity confusion, addiction, and will result in life-long physical, emotional, and social problems.

One rationalization for showing children graphic and even obscene sexual behaviors is to show emotional support for children who might have homosexual or transgender feelings. The assumption is that any child with such feelings must have been "born that way." There is no solid scientific evidence that aberrant sexual behaviors are genetically inherited. "The largest study of its kind…echoes research that says there are no specific genes that make people gay."[201] The same is true for transgender behavior—it is not genetic. To the contrary, there is a great deal of evidence that sexual behaviors are learned. Children who have been molested sexually are much more likely to become molesters themselves. This is learned behavior. Historically, in some cultures all men may engage in bisexual behavior. This is a learned behavior. Cross dressing can be a learned behavior. In this light, schools may be *creating* homosexual and transgender children.

Social Consequences

While the institutionalization of unrestrained sexuality is gaining momentum in K-12 schools, it has already completely taken over our colleges and universities. In the "Emotional Harms" section (above), we saw how Dr. Lisa Wade has explored how unrestrained sexuality has created an "anything-goes" hookup culture on college campuses with its own orgies, rituals, social status, and economics. This is the campus norm. We mentioned earlier a list of colleges and universities that promote unrestrained sexuality through pornography in the classroom. Professors and students who are concerned with what is going on are intimidated and often ridiculed or punished.

Social Harms Summary

The Sexual Holocaust has greatly accelerated the breakdown of key social institutions such as marriage and family. This social harm profoundly amplifies the physical and emotional harm associated with the Sexual Holocaust. The institutions with the most power (the media, the schools, and the government) should be focusing on warning people and society about the dire consequences of unrestrained sexuality. Tragically, they are doing just the opposite. They are glossing over the harmful consequences, while they do everything possible to aggressively promote unrestrained sexuality.

THE SEXUAL HOLOCAUST

In addition to physical, emotional, and social harm, there is a spiritual dimension to the Sexual Holocaust. The spiritual harm of the Sexual Holocaust far outweighs all other harms previously addressed.

CHAPTER 4

HARMFUL SPIRITUAL CONSEQUENCES OF THE SEXUAL HOLOCAUST

There is more sexual freedom today than ever before, with almost everyone, including children, having easy access to every possible type of sexual stimulation. However, more than half the world's people (56%) are unhappy with their sex-life.[202] There is more money spent today on sex-related health care and sex education than ever before. However, pain, disease, addiction, death, depression, suicide rates, divorce, etc., continue to increase with no end in sight. This should tell us that our world is broken, and the cause of this brokenness is fundamentally spiritual. Because the problem is primarily spiritual, mere human efforts are not sufficient to fix the problem.

The vast majority of humans believe there is a spiritual dimension to our lives. As of 2015, 84% of the world identified with a specific religious group. Of the 16% that did not, most were actually NOT atheists. "Some—perhaps most—have a strong sense of spirituality (belief in God, gods or guiding forces), but they don't identify with or practice any organized religion."[203] We may disagree on exactly what the spiritual dimension of humanity looks like, but we almost all agree it is present. In this section, we will look at four spiritual harms of the Sexual Holocaust: (1) Vain or false identities, (2) Guilt and shame, (3) The destruction of true love, and (4) Eternal consequences.

VAIN AND FALSE IDENTITIES

We have already touched on the concept of identity. We looked at how hyper-sexuality places value on sex-appeal and how unrestrained sexual behavior affects identity by making humans into sex-objects. In this section, we will expand on the concept of identity. Much of the current concern about sexual identity is often largely about group membership, personal rights, and pride issues. This includes the presumed spectrum of gender identities, sexual orientations, and the emerging spectrum of new pronouns. In this section, we will discuss three levels of identity: (1) vain identities, those which do not really matter or are fleeting, (2) false identities, those which are not real, and (3) true identities, identities that last.

Vain identities are the way we identity ourselves that are temporary or superficial. Many people, in their desperation, seek identity and worth by trying to create useless or vain personal identities. We may do this by being successful, being cool, belonging to a political party, having unique tattoos, making fashion-statements, belonging to a clique, etc. Because all humans are searching to define themselves, even the shallowest identities (i.e., having certain friends on Facebook), seem to become all-important. However, even good identities can still be vain. Identifying one's self as a teacher or electrician (although those are great careers) is only a temporary identity.

Sexual identity is a vain identity. In a hyper-sexualized world, people seek value through sex-appeal, sexual orientation, declaring certain rights, and a myriad of other concerns. However, each of these is a vain identity. Personal sex-appeal, for example, is temporary, changing, limited, and often subject to someone else's judgement. If human value was based upon sex-appeal, then every baby and every elderly person would have no human value. Likewise, the infirm, disabled, and even seemingly normal people (who don't have bodies like Barbie or Ken) have no value because they don't have sex-appeal. If human value was based upon sexual orientation, then children, and some elderly and disabled individuals would have no value as they may have no sexual interest at all. If people gained their value simply by their political freedoms and rights, then many humans across the world would have no value because they do not actually have rights. Political freedom does not determine whether or not a person has value. Likewise, humans cannot gain their identity and value through their sexuality.

False identities are becoming more and more common. With access to the Internet and social media, anyone can now create a false identity. With large quantities of digital information changing hands, identities can often be hi-jacked. False identities are not just limited to the Internet. Many individuals, who are struggling with their personal value or are having a crisis in their personal identity, want to claim personal identities that are simply not true. For example, some people are claiming ethnicities that do not honestly apply to them. Some even want to identify themselves as non-human ("I am a falcon"). When people claim to be other than what they really are, it can be due to a willful denial of an obvious truth (the belief that truth is personal and people can define their own truth), or it can be delusional (a psychological disassociation from reality).

There are serious gender identity issues associated with rare individuals who suffer from what has for many decades been diagnosed as *gender dysphoria*. This disorder seems to reflect an emotional disconnect between biological reality and a strong desire to become the opposite sex or gender. These people deserve compassion, love, and respect. Studies show that in the long run, cross dressing, hormone treatment, or sex surgery does not generally relieve their emotional distress. They need to discover an identity that is much deeper and truer than mere gender preference, hormone treatments, or sexual surgeries.

We believe the reason for the surge of false identities is because people are desperately searching for their true worth. Humans want purpose, meaning, and value, and when we cannot find it, we make up an identity to fill the void. However, false identities are not truly fulfilling because they are simply not real. We hope that as we seek to understand our true human identity that we can begin to let go of our vain or false identities.

Our research into the unhappy topic of the Sexual Holocaust has been dark; however, we believe there is good news. Our true identity is not temporary or arbitrary. In fact, our identity does not even come from ourselves. We suggest that as humans, our identity comes from God. Humans were *created in the image of God. We are loved by God and have value simply because God chose to give us life*. This type of identity is available to all humanity. No one needs to be excluded. This is a wonderful and lasting identity. It gives us absolute value and worth. We can carry this identity with us wherever we go, for all our lives.

However, with this identity comes responsibility. We are not animals, and, therefore, we need to stop living like animals. God created us as sexual beings, and our sexuality is meant to be sacred. God dictates to us healthy sexual behaviors for our good and gives us a conscience to choose between right and wrong. He also gives us a free will so we can make our own choices. When we try to justify our unrestrained sexual behaviors, we are suppressing our God-given conscience and rejecting our God-given identity. When we do this, we are rejecting what is best for ourselves and others, and instead, we are clinging to selfish pleasures and desires and our vain or false identities. As we will see in the next section, there are serious consequences when we reject our true identity.

GUILT AND SHAME

As we saw earlier in this overview, most unrestrained sexual behaviors are followed by some form of shame, guilt, discomfort, confusion, etc. The inherent guilt that is associated with unrestrained sexual behaviors arises from our conscience and warns us of the multiple harms caused by "anything-goes" sexuality. Guilt is not just associated with the unrestrained sexual behaviors that we physically *do*. It is also associated with what we say and even the sexual thoughts that run through our minds. Being spiritual means that we have the ability to think, reason, and make decisions. Our thoughts are part of who we really are, and we either own them, or they own us.

As we have mentioned, the point of this overview is not for us to judge the behaviors of others; however, it is important to note that those behaviors which cause us and others harm rightfully cause us guilt. It is only reasonable to point out that our sense of guilt is an indicator that a certain behavior is wrong and harmful.

Spiritual Consequences

In some spiritual circles, such behaviors are called sin. Sin causes pain, suffering, and death.

Many institutions are strongly promoting the elimination of negative or convicting words such as sin, guilt, and shame. These things are said to interfere with our happiness and pleasures. However, even if the word "sin" is never spoken, it is still real. We may abolish the word "guilt," but we are still guilty of wrong behaviors. The word "shame" can be forbidden, but we rightfully should still be ashamed of certain behaviors. The push to eliminate words like sin, guilt, and shame is a denial of reality. If people are truly guilty, yet have hardened their hearts and have become truly *shameless*, they cannot be forgiven or healed.

Without acknowledging our wrong behaviors, we have no way to repent or be forgiven. As we normalize irresponsible behaviors in our culture and in our individual lives, our sensitivity changes. We become cold-hearted and spiritually dead. At some point, we can become capable of doing the worst types of evil without even experiencing remorse. If we continue to ignore our consciences, the door to healing can close.

Destruction of True Love

Besides creating false or vain identities and guilt, the Sexual Holocaust is also destroying true love. The ideology being promoted today by the sexual revolution advocates is that "true love always affirms." It affirms all people and all actions. The flip side of that perspective is that anyone who does not affirm all people and all actions is a "hater." However, we suggest that *true love is the exact opposite of the "love" promoted by the sexual revolution.* True love is willing to be restrained because true love puts God and others first.

It should be obvious that not all things should be affirmed. If someone is harming themselves or others, true love would try to intervene. If a minor is starting to use drugs, they should not be affirmed; they should be warned. If a person is dating a sexual predator, they should not be affirmed; they should be warned. If a person wants to change their gender, they should not necessarily be affirmed; they should certainly be warned of the possible harmful physical, emotional, social, and spiritual consequences. True love must be willing to express loving concern, even at the risk of offending someone.

The essence of the Sexual Holocaust is people putting themselves first, before others. Pornography, the hookup culture, sex-trade, abortion, etc. are all examples of individuals seeking their own pleasure above the well-being of others. Selfishness at any cost. People who are championing "anything-goes" sexuality are not showing real love. They are showing universal selfishness. The sexual revolution has replaced real love with sexual acts. However, true love is sacrificial, unconditional, and enduring.

Because we are spiritually broken, we are easily seduced into thinking that personal restraint is a bad thing. Our hearts are not in the right place, and, therefore, it is easy to be persuaded that personal rights should triumph over personal responsibilities.

ETERNAL CONSEQUENCES

The last harm of the Sexual Holocaust is the worst. As we have seen throughout this overview, the Sexual Holocaust ultimately leads to physical, emotional, and social death. Most importantly, it also leads to spiritual death. Since we are given the *ability* to choose between right and wrong and the *freedom* to choose, we will be held *responsible* for our choices. We will be judged for our love (or lack of love) for mankind, and our obedience (or disobedience) toward God.

Most people agree that there is an after-life, and that in the next life there will be consequences. Some people wish to believe there will be no consequences and that we somehow will all just blend together with the cosmos. However, when asked about the most horrible sinners (child molesters or mass murderers), almost all people want to see some type of justice done in the next life. We all want justice. If justice is done in the next life, surely it will be God (not us), who will do the judging. In the end, God is the judge, and we are the judged. Since we will all soon pass-away, this issue should concern everyone.

God dictates to us healthy sexual behaviors for our own good and for the good of those around us. He gave us a conscience to reinforce those truths. However, when we choose to oppose God, we break our relationship with Him, much like an unfaithful spouse who destroys their own marriage. Responsible individuals need to ask themselves if temporary sexual pleasure is worth such an eternal cost.

SPIRITUAL HARMS SUMMARY

Much of humanity has spent the past few decades trying to justify "anything-goes" sexuality. Individuals are increasingly engaging in irresponsible sexual behaviors. As societies become hyper-sexualized, sexuality becomes all-important, and people's identity and value becomes measured by sexual feelings. At the very root of all this pain and suffering is a spiritual conflict. It is now time for us to sober up and acknowledge that we have been going the wrong way. We need to reverse directions. Without God, we cannot win this battle.

At the very heart of all this suffering and evil is a spiritual battle. Instead of trying to justify what we have been doing, we need to admit that unrestrained sexual behaviors are causing profound global harm. We need to stop trying to put a Band-Aid on the symptoms of the Sexual Holocaust, without addressing the cause. We need to realize that the over-arching solution to the crisis is a spiritual revolution that can supersede the sexual revolution. We need to look beyond ourselves to find the answer. Without God, individuals cannot stand against the power behind the Sexual Holocaust. Sexual restraint is a true and responsible manifestation of love.

THE SEXUAL HOLOCAUST SUMMARY

Today, many unrestrained sexual behaviors are permissible and are becoming normalized. These behaviors are being institutionalized, resulting in unspeakable physical, emotional, social, and spiritual harm on a global scale. The sexual revolution has redefined marriage, family, and children and the outcome is a profound breakdown within our society. We have made a commodity out of sex, we have objectified each other, and we are starting to produce designer children. We should not be surprised that loneliness, rejection, depression and suicide are on the rise.

As difficult as these topics are to address, we believe that there are a great number of people who will be able to see the urgency of our message and will join us in urging sexual responsibility and restraint. The cost of ignoring this crisis is unspeakably high. We are paying for this tragedy with our physical health, our emotional health, our social health, and our spiritual health.

THANK YOU

Thank you for reading this overview. It was sobering to write, and we know it was sobering to read. Thank you for your earnest concern for the victims of the Sexual Holocaust. Very likely, various people you care about have been victims of the Sexual Holocaust. Given the magnitude of the problem and given the speed and power of the "sexual tidal wave" that is sweeping across our culture, there is a strong temptation to despair, close our eyes, and shrink back. This temptation to retreat is motivated by self-love, not love for others. At the very least, let us all warn the people we love. Let us at least sound the alarm within the circles where we have some influence. Let our sexual relationships exemplify stable, fulfilling, and committed loving relationships.

WHAT CAN WE DO?

Knowing that money, education and healthcare are not sufficient, what can we do? Certainly we can sound the alarm. Let us encourage one another to do the following:

1. Control/protect our own thoughts, exposures, and behaviors.
2. Encourage loved ones to do the same.
3. Encourage the media to stop exploiting our inherent human sexual vulnerabilities.
4. Encourage social institutions to actively protect children from "anything-goes" sexuality.
5. Encourage governments to label all sexually explicit entertainment as "harmful to public health."
6. Encourage counseling for the purpose of the healing and recovery of sexual victims/addicts.

7. Encourage natural families, as best we can, so children can have a safe and wholesome refuge.
8. Pray that God will change our hearts and rescue us from the power of the Sexual Holocaust.
9. Diligently seek ways to reduce the multiple levels of harm arising from "anything-goes" sexuality.
10. If you have expertise relevant to the four levels of harm (physical, emotional, social, and spiritual), and you share our deep concern, please help us to formulate a global vision of how to stop the spread of the Sexual Holocaust and bring healing to the billions of victims.

For more information, visit:
SexualHolocaust.org

This website will include:
summaries of new developments, useful links,
input from experts who share our concern,
and corrections of our inevitable errors.

APPENDICES

APPENDIX 1 -
Graphs, Charts, and Images

APPENDIX 2 -
Additional Resources

FIGURE 1: FACTORS THAT EFFECT FREQUENCY OF PORNOGRAPHY USE

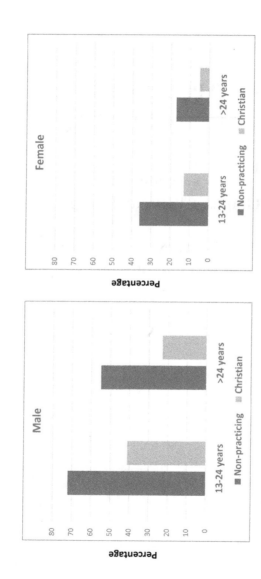

Figure 1 shows that a larger percentage of males (left) use pornography more frequently than females (right). It also shows that a larger percentage of non-practicing Christians (darker shade) use pornography more frequently than practicing Christians (lighter shade). Lastly, it shows that people ages 13-24 use much more pornography than people who are over 24.

APPENDIX 1

FIGURE 2: LEADING CAUSES OF DEATH

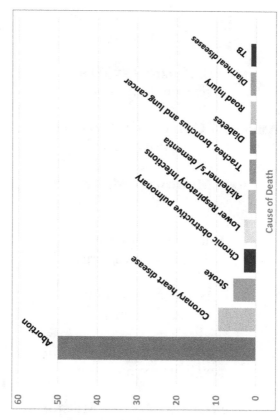

Figure 2 shows the annual number of abortions worldwide (roughly 50 million deaths), compared to the annual top-10 leading causes of death worldwide (the combined total is 34 million deaths).

Appendix 2
Additional Resources

Feed My Sheep Foundation:
fmsfound.org

Sexual Holocaust Website:
sexualholocaust.org

American College of Pediatricians:
acpeds.org

Josh McDowell Ministries:
josh.org

Fight the New Drug:
fightthenewdrug.org

Enough is Enough:
enough.org

Explicit Movement:
explicitmovement.org

International Justice Mission:
ijm.org

World Heath Organization:
who.int

ENDNOTES

INTRODUCTION

1. "Holocaust." Lexico, Powered by Oxford. https://www.lexico.com/en/definition/holocaust.

CHAPTER 1

2. Anonymous. "Heading in a New Direction." TroubledWith. https://www.focusonthefamily.com/lifechallenges/love-and-sex/pornography/heading-in-a-new-direction.

3. "Pornography." Illinois Library. https://guides.library.illinois.edu/c.php?g=347017&p=2341571.

4. Gilkerson, Luke. "Porn 101: College Campuses Using Porn in the Classroom." Covenant Eyes. https://www.covenanteyes.com/2008/10/31/porn-101-college-campuses-using-porn-in-the-classroom/.

5. Fight the New Drug. https://fightthenewdrug.org/.

6. "Pornography." Enough Is Enough. https://enough.org/stats_porn_industry.

7. "Statistics: Porn's Impact on the Brain." Enough Is Enough. https://enough.org/stats-impact-on-the-brain.

8. Weiss, Robert. "Why the Reasons Someone Looks at Porn Matter." Psychology Today. https://www.psychologytoday.com/us/blog/love-and-sex-in-the-digital-age/201607/why-the-reasons-someone-looks-porn-matter.

9. "Mental Effects of Porn." The Reward Foundation: Love, Sex, and the Internet. http://www.rewardfoundation.org/porn-health/mental-effects-of-porn/

10. Ibid.

11. Weiss, Robert. "Why the Reasons Someone Looks at Porn Matter." Psychology Today. https://www.psychologytoday.com/us/blog/love-and-sex-in-the-digital-age/201607/why-the-reasons-someone-looks-porn-matter.

12. "When sex becomes an addiction." CNN. http://www.cnn.com/2008/HEALTH/09/05/sex.addiction/index.html.

13. Bridges, Wosnitzer, Scharrer, Sun, and Liberman. "Aggression and sexual behavior in best-selling pornography videos: a content analysis update." https://www.ncbi.nlm.nih.gov/

pubmed/20980228.

14. "Pornography." Enough Is Enough. https://enough.org/stats_porn_industry.

15. Ibid.

16. Ibid.

17. "Adults & Online Porn." Enough Is Enough. https://enough.org/stats_adults_online_porn.

18. McDowell, Josh. "The Porn Phenomenon Study. Barna Research "Porn in the Digital Age: New Research Reveals 10 Truths." The Porn Epedemic. https://s3.amazonaws.com/jmm.us/PDFs-Downloadable/The+Porn+Epidemic+-+Chapters/The+Porn+Epidemic+-+The+Porn+Phenomenon+Study+(Barna)+-+Updated+1.2019.pdf?iframe=true&width=100%&height=100%%22, 5.

19. Ibid.

20. "Pornography." Enough Is Enough. https://enough.org/stats_porn_industry.

21. McDowell, Josh. "The Porn Epidemic: Extent." https://www.josh.org/resources/apologetics/research/#pornportfolio, 7.

22. BARNA. "Porn in the Digital Age: New Research Reveals 10 Trends." https://www.barna.com/research/porn-in-the-digital-age-new-research-reveals-10-trends/.

23. McDowell, Josh. "The Porn Epidemic." https://www.josh.org/wp-content/uploads/Porn-Epidemic-Executive-Synopsis-9.25.2018.pdf, 11.

24. McDowell, Josh. "The Porn Epidemic, EXTENT." https://www.josh.org/resources/apologetics/research/#pornportfolio, 25.

25. "One in 10 Visitors to Hardcore Porn Sites Is Under 10 Years Old, Study Shows." Fight the New Drug. https://fightthenewdrug.org/data-says-one-in-10-visitors-to-porn-sites-are-under-10-years-old/.

26. "Statistics: Youth & Porn." Enough Is Enough." https://enough.org/stats-youth-and-porn.

27. Ibid.

28. McDowell, Josh. "The Porn Epidemic: Extent." https://www.josh.org/resources/apologetics/research/#pornportfolio, 10.

29. "20 Mind-Blowing Stats About the Porn Industry and Its Underage Consumers." Fight the New Drug. https://fightthenewdrug.org/10-porn-stats-that-will-blow-your-mind/.

30. "Pornography." Enough Is Enough. https://enough.org/stats_porn_industry.

31. McDowell, Josh. "The Porn Epidemic: Extent." https://www.josh.org/resources/apologetics/research/#pornportfolio, 7.

32. "Pornography." Enough Is Enough. https://enough.org/stats_porn_industry.

33. Ibid.

34. Kinnaman, David. The Porn Phenomenon. https://www.barna.com/the-porn-phenomenon/.

35. McDowell, Josh. "The Porn Epidemic: Extent." https://www.josh.org/resources/apologetics/research/#pornportfolio, 8.

36. Ibid.

37. "Pornography." Enough Is Enough. https://enough.org/stats_porn_industry.

38. BARNA. "Porn in the Digital Age: New Research Reveals 10 Trends." https://www.barna.com/research/porn-in-the-digital-age-new-research-reveals-10-trends/.

39. "Drug Abuse and Human Trafficking: Exploring the Connection." The Recovery Village. https://www.therecoveryvillage.com/recovery-blog/drug-abuse-human-trafficking-exploring-connection/#gref.

40. Garcia J., *et al.* "Sexual hook-up culture." American Psychological Association. https://www.apa.org/monitor/2013/02/ce-corner.aspx.

41. Wade, Lisa. *American Hookup.* First Edition. New York, NY. W. W. Norton & Company. 2017, 29-30.

42. Garcia J., *et al.* "Sexual hook-up culture." American Psychological Association. https://www.apa.org/monitor/2013/02/ce-corner.aspx.

43. Wade, Lisa. *American Hookup.* First Edition. New York, NY. W. W. Norton & Company. 2017, 31.

44. Wolf, Naomi. "The Porn Myth." New York. http://nymag.com/nymetro/news/trends/n_9437/.

45. "An Aids orphan's story." BBC News World Edition. http://news.bbc.co.uk/2/hi/africa/2511829.stm.

46. "What Are HIV and AIDS?" HIV Gov. https://www.hiv.gov/hiv-basics/overview/about-hiv-and-aids/what-are-hiv-and-aids.

47. "Antiretroviral HIV Drugs: Side Effects and Adherence." Healthline. https://www.healthline.com/health/hiv-aids/antiretroviral-drugs-side-effects-adherence.

48. Ibid.

49. Sidibé, Michel. "Global HIV and AIDS statistics." Avert. https://www.avert.org/global-hiv-and-aids-statistics.

50. "UNAIDS DATA 2019." https://www.unaids.org/sites/default/

files/media_asset/2019-UNAIDS-data_en.pdf, 16.

51. Sidibé, Michel. "Global HIV and AIDS statistics." Avert. https://www.avert.org/global-hiv-and-aids-statistics.

52. "UNAIDS DATA 2019." https://www.unaids.org/sites/default/files/media_asset/2019-UNAIDS-data_en.pdf, 16.

53. "Sexually transmitted infections (STIs)." World Health Organization. https://www.who.int/news-room/fact-sheets/detail/sexually-transmitted-infections-(stis).

54. "Sexually Transmitted Diseases (STD) Disease-Specific Research." National Institute of Allergy and Infectious Diseases. https://www.niaid.nih.gov/diseases-conditions/std-research.

55. Corlis, Nick. "STI vs. STD." Exposed. https://www.stdcheck.com/blog/std-vs-sti-whats-the-difference/.

56. "HIV in the United States and Dependent Areas." Centers for Disease Control and Prevention. https://www.cdc.gov/hiv/statistics/overview/ataglance.html.

57. "Sexually Transmitted Diseases Control Program." Connecticut State Department of Public Health. https://portal.ct.gov/DPH/Infectious-Diseases/STD/Sexually-Transmitted-Diseases-Control-Program.

58. "Sexually Transmitted Diseases (STD) Disease-Specific Research." National Institute of Allergy and Infectious Diseases. https://www.niaid.nih.gov/diseases-conditions/std-research.

59. "Sexually transmitted infections (STIs)." World Health Organization. http://www.who.int/news-room/fact-sheets/detail/sexually-transmitted-infections-(stis).

60. Ibid.

61. Ibid.

62. Ibid.

63. Ibid.

64. "Statistics." American Sexual Health Association. http://www.ashasexualhealth.org/stdsstis/statistics/.

65. "Sexually transmitted infections (STIs)." World Health Organization. http://www.who.int/news-room/fact-sheets/detail/sexually-transmitted-infections-(stis).

66. "Local African community organizations in Brussels bring attention to children orphaned by AIDS globally." UNAIDS. http://www.unaids.org/en/keywords/orphans.

67. "UNAIDS DATA 2019." https://www.unaids.org/sites/default/files/media_asset/2019-UNAIDS-data_en.pdf, 2.

68. Garcia J., *et al.* "Sexual hook-up culture." American Psychological Association. https://www.apa.org/monitor/2013/02/

ce-corner.aspx.

69. "10 Truly Shocking Stats On STDs and College Students." Nursing Schools. https://www.nursingschools.net/blog/2010/05/10-truly-shocking-stats-on-stds-and-college-students/.

70. "Sexually transmitted infections (STIs)." World Health Organization. http://www.who.int/news-room/fact-sheets/detail/sexually-transmitted-infections-(stis).

71. "India victim in 2012 Delhi gang rape named by mother." BBC News. https://www.bbc.com/news/world-asia-35115974.

72. "Delhi gangrape victim's friend relives the horrifying 84 minutes of December 16 night." India Today. https://www.indiatoday.in/india/north/story/delhi-gangrape-victims-friend-relives-the-horrifying-84-minutes-of-december-16-night-210874-2013-09-13.

73. Barry, Ellen. "In Rare Move, Death Sentence in Delhi Gang Rape Case Is Upheld." The New York Times. https://www.nytimes.com/2017/05/05/world/asia/death-sentence-delhi-gang-rape.html.

74. Tracy, Natasha. "Types of Rape: The Different Forms of Rape." Healthy Place. https://www.healthyplace.com/abuse/rape/types-of-rape-the-different-forms-of-rape.

75. "Consequences of Sexual Assault on the Community." The Advocates for Human Rights. https://www.stopvaw.org/consequences_of_sexual_assault_on_the_community.

76. "Preventing Sexual Violence." https://www.cdc.gov/violenceprevention/pdf/SV-Factsheet.pdf, 1.

77. "FACTSHEET: South Africa's crime statistics for 2018/19." The Citizen. https://citizen.co.za/news/south-africa/crime/2178462/factsheet-south-africas-crime-statistics-for-2018-19/.

78. "Sexual harassment: How it stands around the globe." CNN Health. https://www.cnn.com/2017/11/25/health/sexual-harassment-violence-abuse-global-levels/index.html.

79. Chivers-Wilson, Kaitlin. "Sexual assault and posttraumatic stress disorder: A review of the biological, psychological and sociological factors and treatments." US National Library of Medicine National Institutes of Health. https://www.ncbi.nlm.nih.gov/pmc/articles/PMC2323517/.

80. "Violence against women." World Health Organization. https://www.who.int/news-room/fact-sheets/detail/violence-against-women.

81. Ibid.

82. "Symptoms of Children Who are Victims of Sexual Abuse." Focus on the Family. https://www.focusonthefamily.com/lifechallenges/abuse-and-addiction/sexual-abuse/symptoms-of-children-who-are-victims-of-sexual-abuse.

83. "Human trafficking victim shares story." ICE. https://www.ice.gov/features/human-trafficking-victim-shares-story.

84. "Human Trafficking." Polaris. https://polarisproject.org/human-trafficking?gclid=CjwKCAiAkrTjBRAoEiwAXpf9CZS-3dCjU7Pm_Uag1gy1PJogHqBq8iIfxolmnTMCEPVTzao6eO-EW29xoCBvsQAvD_BwE.

85. Ibid.

86. "Types of Human Trafficking." Human Rights Commission. https://sf-hrc.org/what-human-trafficking#Types of Human Trafficking.

87. Brinlee, Morgan. "13 Sex Trafficking Statistics That Put The Worldwide Problem Into Perspective." Bustle. https://www.bustle.com/p/13-sex-trafficking-statistics-that-put-the-worldwide-problem-into-perspective-9930150.

88. "Drug Abuse and Human Trafficking: Exploring the Connection." The Recovery Village. https://www.therecoveryvillage.com/recovery-blog/drug-abuse-human-trafficking-exploring-connection/#gref.

89. "How Common Is Sex Addiction?" The Ranch Treatment Centers. https://www.recoveryranch.com/resources/sex-addiction-and-intimacy-disorders/sex-addiction-america-common/.

90. Lubin, Gus. "There Are 42 Million Prostitutes In The World, And Here's Where They Live." Business Insider. https://www.businessinsider.com/there-are-42-million-prostitutes-in-the-world-and-heres-where-they-live-2012-1.

91. "Child Abuse Statistics." Invisible Children. http://www.invisiblechildren.org/2017/12/29/child-abuse-statistics-the-best-resources/?gclid=Cj0KCQjwkK_qBRD8ARIsAOteukCz1eSjxoR1hXrF73k7dCvwDjO81J03yBjgfa0tiP3XHDxNSwpuU0waAsGpEALw_wcB.

92. "What is Human Trafficking?" Human Rights Commission. https://sf-hrc.org/what-human-trafficking.

93. "Medical Definition of Induced abortion." Medicine Net. https://www.medicinenet.com/script/main/art.asp?articlekey=17775.

94. Parke, Caleb. "Abortion Survivors on new late-term abortion bills: 'Where were my rights in the womb?'" FOX News.

https://www.foxnews.com/us/abortion-survivors-on-new-late-term-abortion-bills-where-were-my-rights-in-the-womb.

95.   "What Are the Types of Abortion Procedures?" WebMD. https://www.webmd.com/women/abortion-procedures#1.

96.   "Aspiration Abortion." Abortion Procedures. https://www.abortionprocedures.com/aspiration/#1466797068169-b19ae05d-8be7.

97.   "Fact Sheet: Science of Fetal Pain." Charlotte Lozier Institute. https://lozierinstitute.org/fact-sheet-science-of-fetal-pain/.

98.   "D & E Abortion." Abortion Procedures. https://www.abortionprocedures.com/#1466802056779-57286d5b-0d60.

99.   "Induction Abortion." Abortion Procedures. https://www.abortionprocedures.com/induction/#1466802482689-777ef64c-4991.

100.   "Abortion Complications." Focus on the Family. https://www.focusonthefamily.com/socialissues/life-issues/dignity-of-human-life/abortion-complications.

101.   Lisa B. Haddad, and Nawal M. Nour. "Unsafe Abortion: Unnecessary Maternal Mortality." US National Library of Medicine National Institutes of Health. https://www.ncbi.nlm.nih.gov/pmc/articles/PMC2709326/.

102.   "U.S. Abortion Statistics." Abort73. https://abort73.com/abortion_facts/us_abortion_statistics/.

103.   http://www.jpands.org/vol22no4/coleman.pdf

104.   "U.S. Abortion Statistics." Abort73. https://abort73.com/abortion_facts/us_abortion_statistics/.

105.   "Maternal mortality." World Health Organization. https://www.who.int/news-room/fact-sheets/detail/maternal-mortality.

106.   "U.S. Abortion Statistics." Abort73. https://abort73.com/abortion_facts/us_abortion_statistics/.

107.   Mitchell, Tony. "The leading causes of death in the world - can they be cured?" Proclinical. https://www.proclinical.com/blogs/2017-5/the-leading-causes-of-death-in-the-world-can-they-be-cured

108.   "Number of Abortions - Abortion Counters." http://www.numberofabortions.com/.

CHAPTER 2

109.   "Porn is Inspiring Teen Girls to Undergo This Invasive and Painful Cosmetic Surgery." Fight the New Drug. https://fight-

thenewdrug.org/growing-trend-of-porn-inspired-plastic-sur-gery-for-teens/.

110. "Porn Star Surgery...aka "The Barbie." Medical Bag. https://www.medicalbag.com/home/features/body-modification/porn-star-surgeryaka-the-barbie/.

111. "Porn is Inspiring Teen Girls to Undergo This Invasive and Painful Cosmetic Surgery." Fight the New Drug. https://fight-thenewdrug.org/growing-trend-of-porn-inspired-plastic-sur-gery-for-teens/.

112. Wolf, Naomi. "The Porn Myth." New York. http://nymag.com/nymetro/news/trends/n_9437/.

113. Peirce, Andrea. "The Emotional Impact of an HIV Diagnosis." Everyday Health. https://www.everydayhealth.com/hiv-aids/hiv-diagnosis-emotional-impact.aspx.

114. "How many adults have STDs/STIs?" PLUS. https://www.hivplusmag.com/prevention/2015/09/25/shock-ing-stats-stds-america?pg=1#article-content.

115. Boskey, Elizabeth. "How STDs Can Play a Role in Abusive Relationships." Verywell Health. https://www.verywell-health.com/how-stds-can-play-a-role-in-abusive-relation-ships-3132706.

116. Corlis, Nick. "STDs and The Law." Exposed. https://www.stdcheck.com/blog/stds-and-the-law/.

117. "What is PTSD?" The Meadows. https://www.themeadows.com/conditions-we-treat/post-traumatic-stress-disorder/.

118. "Dissociation." RAINN. https://www.rainn.org/articles/dissoci-ation.

119. "Self-harm." RAINN. https://www.rainn.org/articles/self-harm.

120. "The Emotional Side Effects of Abortion." Unplanned Pregnancy Association. http://americanpregnancy.org/un-planned-pregnancy/abortion-emotional-effects/.

121. Coleman P. K., *et al.* 2017. Women Who Suffered Emotionally from Abortion: A Qualitative Synthesis of Their Experiences. Journal of American Physicians and Surgeons. 22 (4): 113-118.

122. Yoder, Katie. "Media Hide New Research on Women Harmed by Abortion." Catholic Citizens. https://catholiccitizens.org/views/77115/media-hide-new-research-women-harmed-abor-tion/.

123. Ibid.

124. Carlton, Kat. "What is loneliness?" UChicago Medicine. https://www.uchicagomedicine.org/forefront/health-and-well-ness-articles/2019/february/what-is-loneliness.

125. Wolf, Naomi. "The Porn Myth." New York. http://nymag.com/nymetro/news/trends/n_9437/.

126. Schulze, Hannah. "Loneliness: An Epidemic?" Harvard University. http://sitn.hms.harvard.edu/flash/2018/loneliness-an-epidemic/.

127. Ibid.

128. "Top 10 Most Common Human Fears and Phobias." Learning Mind. https://www.learning-mind.com/top-10-most-common-human-fears-and-phobias/.

129. LaFee, Scott. "Serious Loneliness Spans the Adult Lifespan but there is a Silver Lining." UC San Diego Health. https://health.ucsd.edu/news/releases/Pages/2018-12-18-Serious-Loneliness-Spans-Adult-Lifespan-but-there-is-a-Silver-Lining.aspx.

130. Lardieri, Alexa. "Study: Many Americans Report Feeling Lonely, Younger Generations More So." U.S. News. https://www.usnews.com/news/health-care-news/articles/2018-05-01/study-many-americans-report-feeling-lonely-younger-generations-more-so.

131. Ibid.

132. Justin R. Garcia, Chris Reiber, Sean G. Massey, and Ann M. Merriwether. "Sexual hook-up culture." American Psychological Association. https://www.apa.org/monitor/2013/02/ce-corner.aspx.

133. Wade, Dr. Lisa. American Hookup. First Edition. New York, NY. W. W. Norton & Company. 2017, 36.

134. Wade, Dr. Lisa. American Hookup. First Edition. New York, NY. W. W. Norton & Company. 2017, 14.

135. Eisenberger, Lieberman, and Williams. "Does rejection hurt? An FMRI study of social exclusion." US National Library of Medicine National Institutes of Health. https://www.ncbi.nlm.nih.gov/pubmed/14551436.

136. Winch, Guy. "10 Surprising Facts About Rejection." Psychology Today. https://www.psychologytoday.com/us/blog/the-squeaky-wheel/201307/10-surprising-facts-about-rejection.

137. Ibid.

138. Weir, Kirsten. "The pain of social rejection." American Psychological Association. https://www.apa.org/monitor/2012/04/rejection.

139. Winch, Guy. "10 Surprising Facts About Rejection." Psychology Today. https://www.psychologytoday.com/us/blog/the-squeaky-wheel/201307/10-surprising-facts-about-rejection.

140. "Depression Basics." National Institute of Mental Health.

https://www.nimh.nih.gov/health/publications/depression/index.shtml.

141. "What causes depression?" Harvard Health Publishing. https://www.health.harvard.edu/mind-and-mood/what-causes-depression.

142. Ibid.

143. Nemade, Rashmi. "Depression: Depression & Related Conditions." Gulf Bend Center. https://www.gulfbend.org/poc/view_doc.php?type=doc&id=13010&cn=5.

144. Alexa Negele, Johannes Kaufhold, Lisa Kallenbach, and Marianne Leuzinger-Bohleber. "Childhood Trauma and Its Relation to Chronic Depression in Adulthood." US National Library of Medicine National Institutes of Health. https://www.ncbi.nlm.nih.gov/pmc/articles/PMC4677006/.

145. Ibid.

146. Morin, Amy. "Depression Statistics Everyone Should Know." Verywell Mind. https://www.verywellmind.com/depression-statistics-everyone-should-know-4159056.

147. Alexa Negele, Johannes Kaufhold, Lisa Kallenbach, and Marianne Leuzinger-Bohleber. "Childhood Trauma and Its Relation to Chronic Depression in Adulthood." US National Library of Medicine National Institutes of Health. https://www.ncbi.nlm.nih.gov/pmc/articles/PMC4677006/.

148. Fox, Maggie. "Major depression on the rise among everyone, new data shows." NBC News. https://www.nbcnews.com/health/health-news/major-depression-rise-among-everyone-new-data-shows-n873146.

149. "Suicide." World Health Organization. https://www.who.int/news-room/fact-sheets/detail/suicide.

150. Ibid.

151. Ibid.

152. "Suicide data." World Health Organization. https://www.who.int/mental_health/prevention/suicide/suicideprevent/en/.

153. Ibid.

154. Ibid.

CHAPTER 3

155. Kim Parker and Renee Stepler. "As U.S. marriage rate hovers at 50%, education gap in marital status widens." Pew Research Center. https://www.pewresearch.org/fact-tank/2017/09/14/

as-u-s-marriage-rate-hovers-at-50-education-gap-in-marital-status-widens/.

156. Ibid.

157. "Which EU countries have the highest marriage rates?" EuroStat. https://ec.europa.eu/eurostat/web/products-eu-rostat-news/-/EDN-20190214-1?inheritRedirect=true.

158. Steger, Isabella. "People don't want to get married in South Korea anymore." Quartz. https://qz.com/1234031/marriages-and-birth-rate-in-south-korea-fall-to-record-lows-according-to-census-statistics/.

159. Sharma, Neetu Chandra. "Non-marriage very rare in India but divorces doubled in past two decades." LiveMint. https://www.livemint.com/news/india/non-marriage-very-rare-in-india-but-divorces-doubled-in-past-two-decades-report-1561486297890.html.

160. LaScala, Marisa. "The U.S. Divorce Rate Is Going Down, and We Have Millennials to Thank." Good Housekeeping. https://www.goodhousekeeping.com/life/relationships/a26551655/us-divorce-rate/.

161. "Supreme Court unravels definition of marriage." The Family Leader. https://thefamilyleader.com/supreme-court-unravels-definition-of-marriage/.

162. Nelson, Steve. "'Sister Wives' Defeat Polygamy Law in Federal Court." U.S. News. https://www.usnews.com/news/articles/2013/12/16/sister-wives-defeat-polygamy-law-in-federal-court.

163. Mince-Didier, Ave. "Incest Laws and Criminal Charges." Criminal Defense Lawyer. https://www.criminaldefense-lawyer.com/resources/criminal-defense/white-collar-crime/incest-laws-criminal-charges.htm.

164. Syrett, Nicholas. "Child marriage is still legal in the US." The Conversation. http://theconversation.com/child-marriage-is-still-legal-in-the-us-88846.

165. Wisch, Rebecca. "Table of State Animal Sexual Assault Laws." Michigan State University. https://www.animallaw.info/topic/table-state-animal-sexual-assault-laws.

166. "How Porn & Technology Might Be Replacing Sex for Japanese Millennials." Fight the New Drug. https://fightthe-newdrug.org/how-porn-sex-technology-is-contributing-to-ja-pans-sexless-population/.

167. "EXCLUSIVE: Futurologist Dr. Ian Pearson On Sex With Robots, Contact Lens VR, And More." BREITBART.

https://www.breitbart.com/tech/2016/07/05/exclusive-people-will-emotional-sex-robots-2030-according-futurologist-dr-ian-pearson/.

168. "Sex Robots Are Becoming A Reality, But Are They Dangerous For Society?" Fight the New Drug. https://fightthenewdrug.org/futurologist-says-sex-with-robots-will-become-reality-by-2050/.

169. Ibid.

170. Jozuka, Emiko. "Japan suffers biggest natural population decline ever in 2018." CNN Health. https://www.cnn.com/2018/12/23/health/japan-birthrate-record-low-intl/index.html.

171. Semuels, Alana. "The Mystery of Why Japanese People Are Having So Few Babies." The Atlantic. https://www.theatlantic.com/business/archive/2017/07/japan-mystery-low-birth-rate/534291/.

172. "How Porn & Technology Might Be Replacing Sex for Japanese Millennials." Fight the New Drug. https://fightthenewdrug.org/how-porn-sex-technology-is-contributing-to-japans-sexless-population/.

173. "South Korea's population crisis worsens as its fertility rate plummets to record low." South China Morning Post. https://www.scmp.com/news/asia/east-asia/article/2187974/south-koreas-population-crisis-worsens-its-fertility-rate.

174. Wallerstein, Judith. "The Long-Term Effects of Divorce on Children: A Review." Science Direct. https://www.sciencedirect.com/science/article/abs/pii/S0890856709645500.

175. Pickhardt, Carl. "The Impact of Divorce on Young Children and Adolescents." Psychology Today. https://www.psychologytoday.com/us/blog/surviving-your-childs-adolescence/201112/the-impact-divorce-young-children-and-adolescents.

176. Ibid.

177. Manning, Wendy. "Cohabitation and Child Wellbeing." US National Library of Medicine National Institutes of Health. https://www.ncbi.nlm.nih.gov/pmc/articles/PMC4768758/.

178. Ibid.

179. DeRose, Laurie. "Cohabitation Contributes to Family Instability Across the Globe." Institute for Family Studies. https://ifstudies.org/blog/cohabitation-contributes-to-family-instability-across-the-globe.

180. Therese Hesketh and Zhu Wei Xing. 2006. "Abnormal sex ratios in human populations: Causes and consequences." US

National Library of Medicine National Institutes of Health. https://www.ncbi.nlm.nih.gov/pmc/articles/PMC1569153/. PNAS. 103(36): 13271-13275.

181. Ibid.
182. Ibid.
183. Ibid.
184. Ibid.
185. Ibid.
186. Ibid.
187. Ibid.
188. "Abortion Bans in Cases of Sex or Race Selection or Genetic Anomaly." Guttmacher Institute. https://www.guttmacher.org/state-policy/explore/abortion-bans-cases-sex-or-race-selection-or-genetic-anomaly.
189. Ibid.
190. Somarriba, Mary Rose. "The Overlooked Risks of Surrogacy for Women." Institute for Family Studies. https://ifstudies.org/blog/the-overlooked-risks-of-surrogacy-for-women.
191. Ibid.
192. Carroll, Linda. "New study tracks emotional health of 'surrogate kids.'" Today. https://www.today.com/health/new-study-tracks-emotional-health-surrogate-kids-6C10366818.
193. "West Coast Surrogacy Costs & Fees." West Cost Surrogacy. https://www.westcoastsurrogacy.com/surrogate-program-for-intended-parents/surrogate-mother-cost.
194. "Surrogacy in the United States." The Sensible Surrogacy Guide. https://www.sensiblesurrogacy.com/surrogacy-in-the-united-states/.
195. "Heritable genome editing: action needed to secure responsible way forward." Nuffield Council on Bioethics. http://nuffieldbioethics.org/news/2018/heritable-genome-editing-action-needed-secure-responsible.
196. "Genome damage from CRISPR/Cas9 gene editing higher than thought." Science Daily. https://www.sciencedaily.com/releases/2018/07/180719165032.htm.
197. Ibid.
198. Stein, Rob. "Chinese Scientist Says He's First To Create Genetically Modified Babies Using CRISPR." NPR. https://www.npr.org/sections/health-shots/2018/11/26/670752865/chinese-scientist-says-hes-first-to-genetically-edit-babies.
199. Satyajit Patra and Araromi Adewale Andrew. "Human, Social, and Environmental Impacts of Human Genetic Engineering."

Journal of Biomedical Sciences. http://www.jbiomeds.com/
biomedical-sciences/human-social-and-environmental-im-
pacts-of-human-genetic-engineering.php?aid=7264.

200. Morrar, Sawsan. "Porn or vital life lessons? California ap-
      proves controversial new sex education curriculum." MSN.
      https://www.msn.com/en-us/news/us/porn-or-vital-life-les-
      sons-california-approves-controversial-new-sex-education-cur-
      riculum/ar-AAB7wux?ocid=spartanntp.

201. "A 'gay gene'? It's complicated, according to new research on
      same-sex behavior." NBC News. https://www.nbcnews.com/
      feature/nbc-out/new-genetic-links-same-sex-sexual-behavior-
      found-n1047951.

CHAPTER 4

202. "Give and receive 2005 Global Sex Survey result." Data360.
      http://www.data360.org/pdf/20070416064139.Global%20
      Sex%20Survey.pdf.

203. Sherwood, Harriet. "Religion: why faith is becoming more and
      more popular." The Guardian. https://www.theguardian.com/
      news/2018/aug/27/religion-why-is-faith-growing-and-what-
      happens-next.